NS-05

Vital Notes for Nurses:
Accountability

For Brian, for always

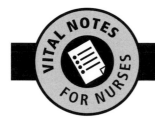

VITAL NOTES FOR NURSES

Accountability

Helen Caulfield
Solicitor, LLB, MA, MSc

Blackwell
Publishing

Blackwell Publishing Ltd
Editorial offices:
Blackwell Publishing Ltd, 9600 Garsington Road, Oxford OX4 2DQ, UK
    Tel: +44 (0)1865 776868
Blackwell Publishing Inc., 350 Main Street, Malden, MA 02148-5020, USA
    Tel: +1 781 388 8250
Blackwell Publishing Asia Pty Ltd, 550 Swanston Street, Carlton, Victoria
3053, Australia
    Tel: +61 (0)3 8359 1011

First published 2005 by Blackwell Publishing Ltd

Library of Congress Cataloging-in-Publication Data
is available

ISBN-10: 1-4051-2279-X
ISBN-13: 978-1-4051-2279-5

A catalogue record for this title is available from the British Library

Set in 10/12 pt Palatino
by SNP Best-set Typesetter Ltd., Hong Kong
Printed and bound in Great Britain
by TJ International Ltd, Padstow, Cornwall

The publisher's policy is to use permanent paper from mills that operate a
sustainable forestry policy, and which has been manufactured from pulp
processed using acid-free and elementary chlorine-free practices. Further-
more, the publisher ensures that the text paper and cover board used have
met acceptable environmental accreditation standards.

For further information on Blackwell Publishing, visit our website:
www.blackwellnursing.com

Contents

Preface

This introductory text sets out a framework for accountability. It is intended to show that law, ethics, employment and professional issues are complementary in nursing practice. Taken together, they form a framework against which clinical issues can be considered.

The book sets out the four pillars of accountability, and considers the structures, rights and redress of the health service. There are two detailed chapters on the concepts of negligence and consent. Application of the framework is then made in the key area of confidentiality, and in a final chapter applied also to two examples that are often contentious in nursing practice: termination of pregnancy and dying. The purpose is to set out a systematic approach and demonstrate how this can be applied to any area of nursing practice.

I have worked for nurses for over a decade, and my passion has always been to demystify the law for nurses. That wonderful sound 'aha!' when an individual or a conference of nurses suddenly realises the law is straightforward at its heart will always be my goal. As nurses gain confidence in the key principles that shape the clinical relationship, the quality of care that is given to patients and clients can only be improved.

As I have developed this framework over the past four years I have had considerable feedback from many nurses, and I am indebted to all those who have helped me expand and refine this work. Particular thanks go to my colleagues, past and present, in the legal, policy and nursing practice departments at the Royal College of Nursing from whom I never cease learning.

Any errors or omissions in this text are of course my own responsibility.

Helen Caulfield

A Framework of Accountability for Nurses

Learning objectives

This chapter sets the scene for the whole text. It describes the basic framework of accountability that can be used in all areas of nursing practice. The framework is made up of four pillars of accountability: professional, ethical, legal and employment. This framework is the key to understanding the four pillars of accountability, and their inter-relationship with each other. Taken together, they provide a complete framework of accountability for nursing practice.

The learning objectives for this chapter are to:

- understand the framework of accountability
- assess the four pillars of accountability in nursing practice
- identity the source of each of pillar of accountability
- place each pillar of accountability in the context of nursing practice
- apply the framework to real examples of nursing practice
- consider further issues arising in each example using the framework
- be confident that the framework applies to every part of nursing practice.

Introduction

It is possible that there was a time when a single source of nursing practice accountability existed. This would have meant that nurses, patients, managers, the media, government and your next door neighbour all had exactly the same understanding of what was expected from a nurse.

Today it is universally clear that there is no single source of accountability for nurses; the different types of accountability for nursing practice come from an increasing range of sources. This may be from a regulatory perspective, particularly the Nursing and Midwifery Council (NMC). It may be from a legal perspective, either from legislation or from court judgments. It may be from the media, where the headlines of the day shape the overall impression of the profession of nursing. It may be from the range of agencies and government departments that send out directions and guidance to managers who in turn ask that nurses translate this into their employment practice. As a result, there are many different sources of accountability in nursing practice. Being aware of each type of accountability and the way it affects practice can be a complex issue. Where do you start?

Different bodies set standards for health care or nursing practice and they each require different levels of responsibility from nurses. Sometimes this means that nurses have to take specific action, or that nurses have to be aware of the minimum standards that are in place in the health setting in which they work. Because each body has different standards, there are different penalties they can impose if the standards that create accountability are not met. This chapter sets out in broad terms the authority, standards and penalties of each authority. The framework of accountability ensures that all these sources of authority are easy to characterise and ensures that accountability can be applied in all areas of nursing practice.

Summary

- There are many different sources of accountability.
- There is no single source of accountability for nurses.
- Different authorities create structures and standards.
- Different bodies can impose penalties on nursing practice.
- A framework of accountability gives consideration to these standards.
- This will provide a system that is easy to characterise and can be used in all areas of nursing practice.

A framework of accountability

Many nurses will ask 'am I accountable for this?' when they reach a point of tension in their relationships with patients, with other health care professionals and sometimes with their employers. This is a valid question whenever this tension arises. The consideration of what accountability means in nursing practice is a key part of the foundation of nursing.

Some would say that being accountable means being responsible, and as a consequence taking the blame when something goes wrong. This approach to accountability reduces its scope and may lead to defensive nursing practice. This happens when nurses are worried that they may be singled out for criticism. Defensive practice may lead to an overreliance on protocols at the expense of clinical judgement. It may happen where the safest option is chosen for the patient, even though a newer approach may lead to better health outcomes.

A wider view of accountability is that it is an inherent confidence as a professional that allows a nurse to take pride in being transparent about the way he or she has carried out their practice. It requires that nurses make informed decisions about what approach to use. It means that nurses engage with clients and patients to agree on a joint approach with confidence and assurance.

This book is based on a framework of accountability that considers approaches based on four pillars that set out different types of authority in nursing practice:

- professional
- ethical
- law
- employment.

This chapter summarises the main issues under each of these four pillars. Each pillar then has its own chapter so that a more detailed assessment of the framework of accountability can be given.

Summary

- Nurses have different ways of understanding accountability.
- Some nurses think being accountable is the same as being blamed.
- Others think being accountable is being responsible for the actions of others.
- Defensive practice can arise if nurses believe being accountable is the same as being blamed.
- Some believe being accountable is the distinguishing mark of a profession.
- A professional who is accountable can be confident and assured.
- Nurses have to respond to different types of authority.
- All these authorities provide a collective sense of accountability.
- This framework of accountability is made up of four pillars: professional, ethical, legal and employment.
- The four pillars of accountability are set out in general terms in this chapter.
- Each pillar of accountability is described in more detail in individual chapters.

- Areas of specific nursing practice are set out in detail in later chapters with a close assessment of their relationship with the framework of accountability.

Activity

What does being accountable mean to you as an individual? Write down the influences that have lead you to this view.

Ask your colleagues at work what they think being accountable means. Does this change your mind?

Keep a note of the responses at this stage. When you reach the end of this book, repeat this activity and see if your responses have altered.

The first pillar of accountability: professional accountability

Professional accountability is at the heart of nursing practice. This consists of an ethos in nursing that is based on promoting the welfare and wellbeing of patients through nursing care. Professional accountability allows nurses to work within a framework of practice and to follow principles of conduct that maintain the patient's trust in the individual nurse and support for the nursing profession as a whole.

This drive to demonstrate professional accountability led to the creation of a body that was responsible for setting the standards of conduct and practice for nurses. This is the regulatory body for nurses and midwives. It has taken on different names over the last hundred years, and is currently the Nursing and Midwifery Council (NMC).

One of the functions of the NMC is to create the limits on professional accountability in nursing and midwifery practice. The most obvious way that the NMC does this is by publishing the Code of Professional Conduct (NMC, 2002). This covers all nurses and midwives who are on the register.

The NMC Code of Professional Conduct clause 1.3 states that 'you are personally accountable for your practice. This means that you are answerable for your actions and omissions, regardless of advice or directions from another professional.'

The NMC may publish other standards or guidance for those on the register. These also form part of the framework of professional accountability for nurses and midwives. This is a personal relationship between the nurse and the regulator that cannot be delegated to another person.

Summary

- Professional accountability creates a framework of practice.
- Professional accountability creates principles of conduct.

- The body that sets standards for nurses has existed for nearly a century.
- This body is now known as the Nursing and Midwifery Council (NMC).
- The NMC sets limits on professional accountability in nursing practice.
- The NMC Code of Professional Conduct provides the minimum standard of professional behaviour required from nurses and midwives.
- The NMC Code of Professional Conduct is personal to every nurse or midwife.
- The relationship between the nurse or midwife and the NMC is a personal relationship, and cannot be delegated to another nurse or midwife.

Case study 1.1: Professional accountability

Sally Ann is a staff nurse in an oncology unit. She has been registered with the NMC since she qualified in 1998. She is well regarded at work and is in line for a promotion. She has been so busy at work that she has put off updating her portfolio, and she has not attended any study days. When it is time for her to re-register with the NMC, she realises that she has not completed her continuing professional development (CPD) requirements.

What do you think are the main issues for Sally Ann in her professional accountability at this stage?

Sally Ann decides to lie about her continuing education. She completes the form for the NMC and states that she has completed the minimum requirements for continuing professional development.

Does this change the main issues in professional accountability?

Commentary
The commentary on this case study can be found at the end of the chapter.

Activity

Look at the NMC website (www.nmc-uk.org). There is a section on publications. Which publications set out your limits on accountability? Do you have a copy that is easily to hand for you to reference in your work?

The second pillar of accountability: ethical accountability

Ethical values will form part of the framework of accountability in nursing practice. These ethical values will come from different sources.

Society may have moral constraints on what it is acceptable for a nurse to do in ethical practice. For example, society does not approve of nurses being involved in the torture of individuals. This is a widely held value that is condemned as being against the moral basis of society.

There are other areas in moral codes where society accepts that the practice may be acceptable but recognises that individuals may have their own conscientious objection to participation. The clearest example of this is in relation to termination of pregnancy. While there are limits on the way that a termination can take place, it is recognised that nurses may want to keep a distance from this in their nursing practice.

There will also be ethical practice that the nurse will have for herself. Everyone has their own set of values about the world. Some of these may be based on what they learned at home, at school or in their religious or other community. These values shape the individual approach of the nurse, and it is important that they are reflected in nursing practice. If a nurse has a high value of honesty for herself, it is important that she reflects this in her nursing practice, even where the system of care may not provide the high quality response that her managers would want. Being aware of her personal values will enable the nurse to recognise where these are challenged by different values held by others in nursing practice.

Summary

- Ethical structures are important in health.
- Ethical rules form part of accountability in nursing.
- Ethical accountability may be set by rules decided by society that cover everyone.
- Society may allow conscientious objection to some activity in health care.
- Nurses will have their own moral values that guide their nursing practice.
- Individuals should know their own values and recognise where they are being asked to compromise.

Activity

Take half an hour to consider the personal values that you hold as being essential to who you are as a person. Write down why they are important.

Consider whether your nursing practice incorporates those values. How do you feel when your own values are compromised?

Case study 1.2: Ethical accountability

Annie is a practice nurse in a busy GP practice and has been working there for over seven years. She has completed the Nurse Practitioner course and her qualifications are recorded by the NMC. She runs a series of clinics, including well woman and travel clinics. She reads the travel clinic list for the following day and realises to her horror that one of the clients is a convicted local paedophile. He has recently been released from prison in a blaze of media controversy. She realises that she would be physically revolted at having to provide him with travel vaccinations because her sister was abused as a child.

What do you think are the main ethical issues for Annie at this stage?

Annie speaks about her dilemma to the GP who is not sympathetic to her situation. She decides that she will call in sick the next day, and rings a colleague in another practice who agrees to provide cover for the clinic.

Do her main ethical issues change as a result of her action?

Commentary
The commentary on this case study can be found at the end of the chapter.

The third pillar of accountability: legal accountability

The law is a major area of accountability for nursing practice. The law is a set of rules, regulations and cases that provide interpretation of the rules and regulations which apply in society. There are very clear penalties for anyone, including nurses, where they fail to follow the rules that are set by law.

There are two systems of law in the UK: civil law and criminal law. Each system has its own court structure and different rules apply to each system.

In civil law, the courts will set out the arrangements that apply between private parties. This will include the legal arrangements in areas such as family law, employment law, neighbour disputes and property law, and in areas such as negligence and consent. The types of civil law that will affect accountability in nursing practice include disputes with employers, cases where patients are suing because of allegations of negligence and cases where the nurse sues her employer because she has been injured at work. All these cases are heard in civil courts and the judge can award compensation, which is money to be paid by one side to the other.

In criminal law, the system is designed to assess that rules set by Parliament are followed by every member of society. All law that is criminal has to be set out in an Act of Parliament. If there is no relevant Act of Parliament there can be no criminal activity. The Acts of

Parliament can deal with issues such as medicines, fertility treatment, suicide, organ and tissue donation, mental health and decisions about health care where a person does not have the capacity to make their views known. Criminal penalties include fines or imprisonment.

Summary

- There are two systems of law in the UK: civil and criminal.
- Each system has its own rules and its own court structure.
- Criminal law and civil law are both forms of accountability.
- Both patients and nurses may use either type of law depending on the circumstances of their case.
- Civil law sanctions may involve paying compensation.
- Criminal law sanctions may involve fines or imprisonment.

Case study 1.3: Legal accountability

Gary is a community psychiatric nurse who is stopped by the police for breaking the 30-mile an hour speed limit in a built-up area. He was travelling at 38 miles an hour. He is told that this will be a criminal offence and that he will have 2 points on his driving licence.

What do you think are the main legal issues in this case?

Gary already has 10 points on his licence. This latest traffic offence means that he is about to lose his driving licence completely.

Do the legal issues change?

Commentary
The commentary on this case study can be found at the end of the chapter.

Activity

Do you know where to find the name of the lawyer you can turn to when you have a legal issue at work? It might be through your professional organisation or through your employer. Check with both so that you can be clear who you need to contact.

The fourth pillar of accountability: employment accountability

Employers have an important part to play in accountability. Anyone who is employed will have a contract of employment. This is the contractual arrangement. The employed nurse or midwife will see in the contract of employment the duties that they are expected to carry out. They will see details of their pay, the hours they are expected to work and other details which may include a requirement that they remain on the NMC register during their period of employment.

The nurse is accountable to her or his employer. The employer will expect that the duties and responsibilities are carried out safely. The nurse will expect the employer to provide an environment and resources that allow the nurse to carry out her or his contractual duties. The contract of employment will have both explicit and implicit obligations for both the nurse and the employer.

There may be a job description that goes with the contract of employment and this will set out in more detail the role and extent of practice for the nurse. Where the nurse is asked to carry out activities that go beyond the job description, this should be set out in protocols or policies so that the nurse and the employer can be sure that there is agreement about the ways that the job description is being extended.

If the nurse behaves in a way that is not covered by the contract of employment or the job description, the employer has the option of deciding whether to apply some disciplinary measures. This may range from a warning through to a dismissal. If the nurse feels that the employer has acted unfairly, there are employment tribunals that can decide whether the employer should reinstate the nurse or pay her compensation.

Summary

- The employment relationship is another source of accountability.
- The contract of employment sets out the responsibilities and rights for the nurse and the employer.
- Job descriptions may give more detail and set out the extent of the nurse's role.
- Protocols and policies may set out specific activities in the employment relationship.
- Disciplinary measures can be taken by each party in the employment relationship.

Case study 1.4: Employment accountability

Julie is a single mother who works at NHS Direct as a nurse advisor. She only started the job 3 weeks ago, but already has come in late for her shift on more than eight occasions. Her employer calls her for a disciplinary hearing.

What do you think are the main employment issues in this case?

Julie goes to the disciplinary hearing and explains the problems she has juggling the school run with the start time of her shift. She asks whether she can

Continued

work shorter days in term time and longer days during the holidays. Her employer says this is not possible. Julie decides to stay in this post.
What employment issues change as a result?

Commentary
The commentary on this case study can be found at the end of the chapter.

Activity

Read your contract of employment and your job description. Where are the limits on accountability that have been set by your employer?

Conclusion

These four pillars of accountability taken together provide a useful framework for all areas of nursing practice. This framework will enable the practitioner to assess where the boundaries are that relate to nursing practice. It will provide clarity about the limits on responsibility in all nursing situations. It will prepare the nurse for a thoughtful assessment of any situation. It will provide answers to the question 'where does accountability exist?' in a lifetime of nursing practice.

By now, you should be able to:
- understand that there are four pillars of accountability in nursing practice
- understand that taken together they form a framework of accountability
- identify the source of each of the pillars of accountability
- place each pillar of accountability in the context of nursing practice
- understand what the powers are for each pillar of accountability
- define the framework of accountability in nursing practice.

Activities

1. Do you think the meaning and limits on accountability in nursing practice will change in the future? What might be the drivers behind such changes?
2. Check websites to see what current text books exist on accountability. Try www.amazon.co.uk as a starting point. Do you think these text books cover every pillar in the framework of accountability?

Commentary on the case studies

Case study 1.1: Professional accountability (see p. 5)

Professional accountability

Sally Ann has not completed her professional educational requirements. She has fallen below the standards required by the NMC and has therefore broken her accountability to her personal regulator. This standard is personal to Sally Ann and cannot be delegated to anyone else. This is her personal responsibility that exists between her and the regulator.

Where the NMC discover that Sally Ann has lied in her information, this would be a matter for the NMC Fitness to Practice procedures. As she made a conscious decision to deceive her regulator, the worst case scenario is that she will be struck off the register. At best, it is likely that a caution would be given by the NMC. This sanction would be declared by the NMC to any current or prospective employer. Members of the public can now search the NMC database and would see this entry.

Ethical accountability

There do not seem to be any aspects of ethical accountability in the first part of this case study. The requirement to complete CPD is a factual aspect of nursing practice.

However, by making a decision to deceive the NMC, Sally Ann has shown that she has values that are not consistent with the regulator. She may gamble that the NMC will never find out, but even if this is the case, she should be aware that her ethical practice is different from the inherent values that would be expected by the NMC.

Legal accountability

There is no legal accountability here. There are no civil or criminal consequences for the failure to complete CPD or for lying to the regulator.

However, if Sally Ann is struck off the register by the NMC for this deception, it becomes a criminal offence to work as a nurse without being on the register. If she is removed from the register, she would be at risk of being prosecuted by the criminal law if she did not tell this to her employer (NMC Order, 2001).

Employment accountability

The failure to complete continuing education may not be a part of the employment contract or the job description. It may depend on the way the contract has been written, and Sally Ann needs to check the provisions. Sally Ann can ask her employer to give her time to complete her CPD so that she can re-register with the NMC.

Continued

If she is removed by the NMC, the employer cannot continue to employ her as a nurse but would be able to employ her as a health care assistant until the situation is resolved.

Case study 1.2: Ethical accountability (see p. 7)

Professional accountability

Annie's ability to provide care in a travel clinic is not in question. She is experienced and competent and would have no difficulty in providing this treatment to any patient. The NMC Code of Conduct does require that she promote the wellbeing of the patient. She may consider that her horror at having to treat him may affect her judgement, and that her nursing skills and the need to provide impartial nursing care may be clouded by her reaction. If this is the case, then her professional accountability is compromised.

Ethical accountability

The key issue here is the ethical accountability for Annie. She recognises that she has a strong personal value that is compromised. This has created a strong personal reaction. She realises that her own personal value system is being challenged by the type of patient she is being asked to treat. She may also recognise that she would have no problem treating the patient if it were a life-saving situation. It may be the fact that the treatment is to enable the patient to travel on holiday that reinforces her sense of revulsion.

Annie's proposed solution is not a clean solution in ethical terms, as Annie has to pretend that she is sick when this is not the case. However, she has made sure that the consequences of her action are covered, and made sure that there is appropriate cover, not just for the patient at the cause of the distress but for all the other patients on her list that day. It has also become clear that her GP does not share the same values as Annie. She may want to consider finding another GP to work for that allows for a discussion about the ethics of the nurse–patient relationship.

Legal accountability

There is no immediate legal accountability here. It is lawful for someone who has been released from a prison sentence to travel and it would be lawful for Annie to provide the vaccinations. The extent to which the patient has to notify the authorities of where he intends to travel is not a matter for Annie. There are no criminal or civil consequences in providing the treatment.

Employment accountability

Part of Annie's contract of employment involves providing the travel clinic and this is also in her job description. Not turning up to the clinic or deciding not to treat a patient where there are no clinical indications may be a breach of her contract.

Case study 1.3: Legal accountability (see p. 8)

Professional accountability
A driving offence is not a matter for the NMC, although the police may notify the NMC that the speeding offence has been recorded. There is no direct impact on patient care, so this is not a breach of the Code of Conduct. If, however, it became clear that there was an underlying reason for the speeding offence, the NMC may want to investigate further. If, for example, the reason Gary was speeding was because he was over the alcohol limit, the NMC may want to be sure that Gary's health was not a matter of concern.

Ethical accountability
There does not seem to be ethical accountability in this case. The speeding offence is a factual matter that has been dealt with by the police.

Legal accountability
The key issue here is legal accountability. Gary has broken the law that covers the maximum speed that can be driven in this area. He has been dealt with by the police for that.

If Gary does lose his licence, it will be because he has already committed other driving offences. It will be important for him to make sure that he contacts his professional body before the hearing into this offence, so that a plea in mitigation can take place for the magistrates to understand what the loss of his driving licence would mean, not just for his work but for his patients. It may be possible for his lawyer to argue that another penalty, such as community service, would be a more practical solution.

Employment accountability
Because Gary is a community nurse and needs to use his car to carry out his employment, there may be employment accountability in this case. Gary will need to notify his employer that he has this criminal record and to assess whether this affects his contract of employment.

Case study 1.4: Employment accountability (see p. 9)

Professional accountability
There may be no professional accountability in this case. Turning up late for work is not a matter for the NMC, particularly where this is as an advisor. It might be a different situation if Julie knew that turning up late would mean that patients were not being provided with nursing care, and did not notify her employer about this on a consistent basis.

Ethical accountability
If the reason for Julie's late arrival at work is related to her domestic situation, it is not immediately apparent that there are ethical issues.

Continued

Legal accountability
There is no apparent legal accountability in this situation. Coming in late to work has no immediate civil or criminal sanctions.

Employment accountability
The key area of accountability here is employment. The employer has the right to expect that staff turn up at the appointed time, and the persistent failure by Julie to do so in a new job would be a matter of concern for the employer.

Julie has not spoken to her employer about the problems of her start time, and waiting for the employer to raise this within the context of a disciplinary hearing will make it much harder for her to negotiate an outcome that suits her. As she has only been employed in the post for a short time, there is a risk that the employer would be able to terminate her contract. If the contract of employment includes a probationary period, this would increase the risk that the employer would terminate her employment at the end of this period without giving reasons.

Useful websites

Institute for Employment Studies: www.employment-studies.co.uk
Nursing Ethics journal: www.nursing-ethics.com
Nursing and Midwifery Council (NMC): www.nmc-uk.org
Legal website links can be found at: www.uk250.co.uk/legal

References

Nursing and Midwifery Council (2002) *Code of Professional Conduct*. NMC, London.
NMC Order. *The Nursing and Midwifery Order 2001*. Statutory Instrument 2002 No 253 Article 44. The Stationery Office, London.

The First Pillar of Accountability: Professional Accountability

Learning objectives

This chapter looks at the role of professional accountability in nursing. It considers the different functions of regulatory bodies for health care, with particular emphasis on the purpose of regulation in health care. It considers the range of professional regulatory bodies, with detailed consideration of the role and activity of the Nursing and Midwifery Council (NMC). It concludes with a view of the future of professional accountability.

The learning objectives in this chapter are to:

- define professional accountability
- place professional accountability in the framework of accountability
- identify the main functions of regulation
- describe the key functions of the Nursing and Midwifery Council
- understand the factors that influence professional accountability
- relate professional accountability across the range of health care settings
- assess what you think is needed to influence professional accountability.

Introduction

The first pillar of accountability is professional accountability. This shapes how the nursing profession is regarded by society. It also defines the standards by which the nursing profession views itself. These standards have been set by the regulators of the individual health professions.

Since the late 1990s, nursing standards can now be set by other national agencies where such standards apply to all professions dealing in a particular aspect of health care. These agencies have a variety of functions, including raising the quality of health care, protecting the public or ensuring safety in practice. Other standards may affect the quality of management in the health system, so that where a nurse is also working as a manager, she or he may need to follow guidance from different sources in achieving professional accountability.

Further guidance that expands the understanding of professional accountability may be provided by different Royal Colleges or professional bodies, which can provide detailed guidance on particular aspects of professional accountability.

Summary

- The first pillar of accountability is professional accountability.
- Professional accountability defines standards for the nursing profession.
- Standards may be set by the profession.
- Professional standards may also be set by national agencies.
- These standards may apply to all health professionals.
- The standards may seek to achieve different results, such as quality or safety.
- Different standards may mean a nurse has to be aware of different sources of professional accountability.
- Further guidance may be given by Royal Colleges and other professional organisations.

A classification of regulation in professional accountability

All parts of the NHS and the independent sector are covered by a system of regulation that relates to people, settings, products and services. In order to create a system of regulation for all these parts of the health service, the Governments in each UK country have created a number of different bodies that set the standards for the service. If these standards are not met, the regulator has powers from the Government to take action.

Regulation is the mechanism by which the Government can influence activity over:

- people
- settings

- products
- services.

People can be regulated in their professional groups by regulators who decide:

- the requirements for entry to that profession
- the circumstances for a person to be removed from the profession
- a Code of Conduct setting out the minimum standards of behaviour expected of those professionals.

Settings can be regulated by agencies of the Government. The Commission for Social Care Inspection in England regulates care homes by a licensing system which sets out the type of care and the number of residents that can be accommodated in each home. The regulations set out minimum standards for the environment of the care home; for example, that each single room must have at least $12\,m^2$ of usable floor space (Department of Health, 2003). If a care home does not comply, it is possible for the licensing body to take away the permission for it to operate as a care home. In extreme cases the regulator can close the health provider.

Products are regulated so that there are standards to ensure that products are fit for purpose. For example, food is regulated in the way that it is packaged and labelled, with use-by dates to guarantee safety. The Government creates agencies that set these standards and inspect to make sure that the standards are being followed. This form of regulation ensures that quality of the product is guaranteed for safety or freshness.

Services are regulated to provide protection for the relationship between the person selling the service and the person buying the service. For example, if you apply for a mortgage you are protected by the Financial Ombudsman Service which sets out the standards that have to be met by the financial advisor. This regulation means that the behaviour of the person providing the service has to be explained at the start of the relationship.

Summary

- The Government regulates people, settings, products and services.
- Regulation is a form of state control on behaviour, environment and quality.
- All parts of society can have different types of regulation.
- Health care has many different forms of regulation.
- Regulatory agencies create minimum standards that are inspected and assessed.
- These agencies set up a licensing system for the provision of a particular service.

- There is power to withdraw the licence if the provider fails to meet the conditions of the licence.

The function of regulation in professional accountability

The UK has seen a rapid growth over the past few years in the creation of different regulatory bodies. These bodies exist to provide performance assessment in improving quality patient care. They also set standards for the health system, both the NHS and the independent sector. The standards have to be followed by the health providers, who are accountable to the regulator in relation to these standards. The penalties if these standards are not followed are that the health provider may receive a negative report, and in some extreme cases may have the management board taken over. Financial penalties may also be imposed.

Each of the regulatory bodies will have a different key function that is their driving force. This may be one of the following:

- improving patient safety
- improving the quality of the health service
- providing national guidelines on treatments for specific illnesses
- monitoring the safety of individuals in the health sector by checking police records
- the management of the service itself.

Each of these regulatory agencies may send teams of inspectors to investigate whether the standards set at a national level are being implemented.

The wide variety of regulatory bodies may create some confusion for nurses in relation to professional accountability. Because each body will want a different type of behaviour or create different reporting mechanisms, there can be an overlap between these agencies in their approach to professional accountability.

Summary

- Different regulatory agencies now exist in each UK country.
- These require standards from the health provider.
- These regulators cover both the NHS and the independent sector.
- Penalties may involve changes to the management of the health provider.
- Inspection is a key mechanism to ensure the standards are being met.
- Nurses need to be clear that in some areas there is overlap.

Case study 2.1: Which regulator?

Ellie is a senior nurse manager in an NHS hospital. She was convicted last month for stealing £3000 of a patient's property. The patient sends a letter of complaint to the NMC asking that an investigation into her fitness to practice takes place. The patient also contacts the Healthcare Commission which regulates the hospital.

The patient has contacted two regulatory bodies, one which covers the regulation of individuals and the other which covers the regulation of settings. Do you think this confuses or complements the accountability of Ellie?

Commentary
The different regulatory bodies assess different functions in the health service. The NMC will assess whether the conviction for theft should have personal consequences for Ellie by a caution or a removal from the register. Given that the primary function of the NMC is public protection, it is likely in this case, where the theft was directly from a patient, that a removal from the register would be the likely outcome.

The Healthcare Commission, on the other hand, will assess whether there was a gap in the systems of the hospital that may need to be assessed on a hospital-wide basis. An investigation of the management of the handling of a patient's property may be triggered by the complaint.

This case illustrates that the same behaviour by a nurse may provoke a different reaction in the regulatory bodies, depending on the function of that regulatory body.

Regulatory bodies for professional accountability

The professional regulatory bodies provide guidance for different professions. These bodies set standards for:

- education for entry to the profession
- a register of those who are competent and fit to practice
- maintaining competence to remain on the register
- discipline, including removing someone from the register on the grounds of misconduct, ill-health or lack of competence.

These regulatory bodies cannot set standards for any profession other than the one that they regulate. The standards that they set for their profession may have an impact on the way that relationships in health care are developed.

The current UK-wide regulators of health care professions are shown in Table 2.1.

Table 2.1   UK-wide regulators of healthcare professions.

Nursing and Midwifery Council	Nurses and midwives
General Medical Council	Doctors
Health Professions Council	13 health professions
Royal Pharmaceutical Society of Great Britain	Pharmacists
General Dental Council	Dentists
General Optical Council	Opticians
General Osteopath Council	Osteopaths
General Chiropractic Council	Chiropractors

The impact of devolution means that, since 1999, any new profession being regulated for the first time can be regulated on a country-by-country basis within the UK (Health Act 1999, section 60). The first example of this new arrangement was social workers, who are now regulated by the body in the country in which they work, including:

• General Social Care Council (England)
• Scottish Social Services Council (Scotland)
• Northern Ireland Social Care Council (Northern Ireland)
• Care Council for Wales (Wales).

Depending on the professional background that applies to a health care worker, each will have to meet the standards in the Code of Conduct for their regulatory body. This is a direct personal relationship that cannot be delegated.

Many health workers are not regulated in this way, including health care assistants and technical staff. New proposals being discussed indicate that regulation of this workforce may take place before 2010.

There is now also an overarching regulatory body for the current UK regulators, the Council for Healthcare Regulatory Excellence (CHRE; formerly the Council for the Regulation of Healthcare Professionals), which was set up by Parliament in the NHS Reform and Health Care Professions Act 2002, section 25. It has the following functions:

• to act as an overarching regulator of people
• to ensure consistency in existing and new health care professions in the UK in areas of practice, discipline and education
• to work with the regulatory bodies so they act in a more consistent manner
• to provide for greater integration and co-ordination between the regulatory bodies
• to promote sharing of good practice and information.

Summary

- There are eight UK-wide regulators for health professions.
- Regulatory bodies set standards for education for the profession.
- There is a register of those who are fit to practice.
- There are standards of practice for each profession.
- These bodies can remove registrants for misconduct, ill-health or lack of competence.
- Since 1999 new professions can be regulated on a country-by-country basis.
- An overarching regulator will streamline the functions of the regulatory bodies.

Activity

A nurse who is removed from the NMC register for striking a patient in anger can work as a health care assistant in the same setting.

Who do you think is the most appropriate regulator for that health care assistant: the NMC, the settings regulator (whether in the NHS or the independent sector) or some other regulator of individuals? What makes you believe this?

Case study 2.2: Regulating the regulators

The NMC heard a case of a nurse who had downloaded pornography from the internet while at work. The NMC issued a caution but decided not to remove the nurse from the register.

The Council for Regulation of Healthcare Professions (CRHP; now the CHRE) wanted to challenge this decision on the grounds that it was 'unduly lenient'. The court had to decide how far the powers of the CRHP could be used in the sentencing powers of the NMC. The Court of Appeal decided that the NMC was in a more expert position to make a judgement about the suitable penalty to impose when a finding of fact that amounted to misconduct had been found.

Commentary
There is some confusion about the extent to which the NMC and other professional regulatory bodies have to assess the quality of their decision making. It is now possible that the CRHP can challenge every decision. The use of the courts is a useful mechanism to assess the extent to which the legislation can be interpreted to decide how the powers of each regulator are used in relation to each other.

CRHP v. *NMC and Truscott* (2004)

The Nursing and Midwifery Council

The regulatory body for nursing has the power to create a register of those nurses and midwives who meet the minimum standards for registration. It also has the power to decide whether to remove an individual from the register for misconduct, lack of competence or ill health. This relationship between the nursing regulator and the individual nurse is personal. It cannot be delegated to anyone else.

The Nursing and Midwifery Council (NMC) is the UK regulatory body for nurses and midwives. It was established in April 2002 by Parliament (NMC Order, 2001). It took over from the former regulator, the United Kingdom Central Council for Nursing, Midwifery and Health Visiting (the UKCC). The NMC is the largest of the UK-wide health regulators.

Summary

- Professional accountability defines standards for the nursing profession.
- The nursing regulator has a personal relationship with the nurse. This cannot be delegated to anyone else.
- The NMC is the largest of the professional regulators.
- The NMC regulates nurses and midwives.
- It was set up in April 2002 and is UK-wide in its authority.

Case study 2.3: NMC health case in fitness to practice

Lisa is a staff nurse who has recently given birth to her third child. Her manager, Joe, has noticed that Lisa has been aggressive with colleagues and forgetful about keeping good nursing records since her return to work. This is not her usual behaviour. Joe wonders whether Lisa may have postnatal depression, but Lisa refuses to see Occupational Health when Joe confronts Her about this. Joe is unsure whether to refer Lisa to the NMC Fitness to Practice process on health grounds. What could Joe do?

Commentary
Joe will need to decide whether a referral after only one conversation with Lisa would justify the process of making a statutory declaration to the NMC. The NMC has published helpful guidance for managers who are concerned about the health of staff and who are thinking of making a referral to the NMC (NMC, 2004a) If Joe does make the referral, he will need to swear a statutory declaration which sets out the behaviour he has seen in Lisa and the action he has taken. The NMC will then ask Lisa to see an independent medical assessor and will hold a hearing at which both Lisa and the medical assessor will be able to

set out whether they believe that Lisa's fitness to practice is impaired. The hearing will be in private and the NMC can decide whether to close the file, keep it open pending further investigation or suspend or remove Lisa from the register.

Activities

1. Look at the NMC website at www.nmc-uk.org and find the details of the most recent fitness to practice case that is reported. Look at the facts of the case and see how the NMC decided to deal with the allegations.
2. Look at the GMC website at www.gmc-uk.org and see how they have reported a case of fitness to practice. Compare this with the way the NMC reports a case. Which case was easier for you to follow and why?

The NMC key functions

The principle functions of the Nursing and Midwifery Council are set out in legislation (NMC Order, 2001), as follows:

- to establish standards of education
- to set up standards of training
- to set up standards of conduct
- to set up standards of performance
- to ensure the maintenance of those standards.

The main objective of the NMC is to safeguard the health and well-being of persons using or needing the services of registrants. The NMC must also have proper regard to the interests of all registrants and prospective registrants in each country of the UK.

A variety of functions must be carried out by the NMC (NMC Order, 2001):

- to create and maintain a register of qualified nurses and midwives
- to set the requirements for evidence of good health and good character
- to create the standards of education and training necessary to achieve the standards of proficiency for entry to the register
- to establish and review the standards of conduct, performance and ethics expected of registrants and prospective registrants and give them such guidance on these matters as it sees fit
- to remove a registrant from the register through the fitness to practice process
- to assess competence and to impose conditions of practice orders.

The overriding objective for the NMC is to safeguard the health and wellbeing of persons using or needing the services of registrants. 'Public protection' is the key mechanism that underpins this.

This is a change from earlier regulatory bodies for nursing and midwifery where the overriding objective was to promote and protect the status of the professions. The NMC does not exist to promote nursing as a career or provide employment or legal advice on an individual basis to nurses. That is the function of the professional bodies such as the Royal College of Nursing and the Royal College of Midwives.

Summary

- The NMC is the largest UK regulator of health professionals.
- Its principal functions are to establish standards for education, practice, conduct and registration.
- Its overriding objective is to provide public protection.
- The NMC has a legal duty to protect the public rather than promote the profession.
- Its objective is to safeguard the health and wellbeing of persons using nursing and midwifery services.

Activity

Look at the functions of the NMC. Do you think these are adequate for the nursing regulator? If you were rewriting the functions, are there any that you would want to add?

Case study 2.4: NMC competence case in fitness to practice

Sunita is an overseas nurse who was admitted to the NMC register after completing an adaptation course in a nursing home. She now works for an NHS Trust in intensive care. The nursing staff are very concerned about her language skills, particularly with the family members of patients. She appears to be abrupt and defensive with them. Also, she does not appear to understand the pressure of the environment and takes a longer time than the other nurses to complete her tasks. How do you think Sunita's competence can be assessed?

Commentary
Since August 2004 the NMC has had the power to assess the competence of an individual nurse. Guidelines have been published to inform managers and members of the public about how the NMC defines competence and the process that will be used to decide whether a nurse lacks competence to the extent that she cannot safely remain on the register (NMC, 2004b).

In Sunita's case it may be, because the environment of intensive care is not what she has been used to, that this is more an issue of adapting to an acute environment rather than of competence. The systems used by the NMC will assess this distinction. It is likely that Sunita will feel pressured as she goes through this process of assessment, and there is a risk that if she lacks confidence in her new setting, this referral will further undermine that confidence. However, this is not the concern of the NMC as their prime function is public protection.

Activity

Go to an NMC fitness to practice hearing. You can find details of where the hearings take place on the website. Make notes of what the surroundings look like and whether they were more or less formal than you expected. Did you understand what the case was about? Who gave evidence and what was the point of the case? Did you feel that the regulator did a good job and why? Did you agree with the decision the panel made? Was the outcome what you expected and why?

The NMC Code of Professional Conduct

In 2002, the NMC published a Code of Professional Conduct (NMC, 2002). The Code is the main source of professional accountability from the NMC for nurses and midwives. It sets out the minimum standard of behaviour expected of a nurse or midwife. Where these minimum requirements are not met, it is possible that the NMC may receive an allegation of unfitness to practise. In extreme cases, the NMC has the power to remove a nurse or midwife from the register.

It is therefore most important that the nurse or midwife has an understanding of the all the requirements of the Code of Conduct at all times of nursing practice. It is important for nurses to be aware of the NMC Code and to notify the regulator in any instance of finding a conflict between their practice and the standards set in the Code.

The NMC Code has a number of sections:

(1) Introduction
(2) Respect the patient as an individual
(3) Obtain consent before any treatment or care
(4) Co-operate with others in the team
(5) Protect confidential information
(6) Maintain professional knowledge and competence
(7) Be trustworthy
(8) Act to identify and minimise the risk to patients and clients.

Where other Codes of Conduct or standards have been set by other bodies, there is a risk that colleagues may be required to act in a way that creates a conflict with the way a nurse is expected to behave. Because of this risk, one of the main tasks for the different regulatory bodies is to ensure that they do not set standards that conflict with the standards of another regulatory body.

Summary

* The main source of nursing professional accountability is the Code of Professional Conduct. This sets out the minimum standards of behaviour required from a nurse.
* Different regulators may set different standards for different health professions.
* Nurses should report to their professional regulator any instance where they find a conflict in different professional standards.

Activities

1. Read the NMC Code of Professional Conduct. Think of a recent difficulty you had at work. Does the Code provide you with guidance so that you are clear what is expected of you? If not, what additional information would you want from the Code?
2. Choose one section from the NMC Code of Professional Conduct. Compare this section with the equivalent extract from the Code of another professional regulatory body. What are the similarities and differences between the sections?

The importance of the NMC in professional accountability

The importance of the NMC for nursing and midwifery accountability is significant. The NMC as regulator sets the boundaries for professional practice. It does so at the minimum level of nursing and midwifery practice. The standards set by the regulator for entry to the register, for example, are the minimum standards that an individual must achieve in order to be allowed to practise safely as a nurse or midwife. In addition, the NMC will be setting standards for regulating advanced nursing practice so that the public can be sure that a nurse who claims to be working at an advanced level is being regulated in this by the NMC. In addition, the NMC can record specific aspects of nursing practice. At present, this covers those nurses who have asked to be recorded as nurse prescribers.

The NMC has to keep a register and make sure that those admitted to the register have achieved the right levels of educational and practical expertise. The NMC also has to ensure that each person on the register satisfies their requirements for good health and good character. Once a person is on the register they have to re-register every three years and achieve minimum requirements for continuing professional development.

The registrants pay for registration, which provides them with the licence to practise as a nurse or a midwife. If an individual is not on the register, it is a criminal offence for her or him to pretend to be a registered nurse (NMC Order, 2001, Article 44).

Summary

- The NMC sets minimum standards for registration.
- The NMC has to keep a register of all nurses and midwives who are able to practise.
- It is a criminal offence to pretend to be on the register.

Case study 2.5: The balance of public protection

A nursing home owner referred the matron to the police. The police interviewed the nurse but decided to take no further action. The nursing home owner referred the matron to the previous nursing regulator, the UKCC. The UKCC wanted a copy of the tape recorded interview held by the police. The nurse refused to give permission for the tapes to be given to the UKCC.

The case went to court, where the issue to be decided was whether the public protection interest of the UKCC was more important than the nurse's right to keep her interview confidential with the police. The Court of Appeal decided that the public protection role of the UKCC was more important. Because the UKCC had the power to remove a nurse from the register, the court decided that this investigation could include a request by the UKCC to see police interview material. This was even where the police decided that no criminal activity had taken place.

Commentary
When a nurse gives evidence to the police she needs to be aware that her statement or the tape recording of her interview can be called for by the NMC in the event that an allegation of fitness to practice is made. Nurses need to be aware when they assist the police that other regulators may then ask for that information.

Woolgar v. *Chief Constable Sussex Police and UKCC* (1999)

Other codes of conduct and guidance

The professional standard of accountability set by the NMC covers nursing and midwifery. When you work with another health professional, he or she will have a professional standard of accountability that may differ from your professional standards. For example, the General Medical Council (GMC) is the body that regulates doctors. It has a set of standards for doctors that create the limits on professional accountability (GMC, 2001).

There may be other Codes of Conduct that will have an effect on the overall accountability of nurses. For example, the NHS in England has a Code of Practice for Managers that will cover all nurses who work as managers in the NHS (Department of Health, 2002). This does not have penalties if the content of the Code has been broken. Where a nurse manager does not follow the NHS Code, she may find it hard to get another job as an NHS manager, but where a nurse or midwife does not follow the NMC Code, she is at risk of being struck off the register. So where a nurse is a manager and breaks some aspect of each Code, the NMC Code can impose a more stringent sanction than the NHS Code.

Professional organisations may set standards for accountability in a particular area of nursing practice. For example, the Royal College of Physicians has published guidance on diagnosis and management of patients in a vegetative state (RCP, 2003). Nurses working in this area need to know the current standards for this specialised area, even though the standards are not set by their own professional body.

Summary

- All regulated health professions have their own Code of Practice.
- These Codes of Practice may differ from each other.
- Codes of Conduct may apply to nurses even when they are not published by the NMC.
- Guidance from professional organisations can create standards for accountability.

Activity

Your hospital has problems with its catering contract. Very often the food is not hot by the time it reaches the patients. An earlier Healthcare Commission report criticised standards of nutrition. You are aware that all members of the team are frustrated by pressure to keep to a strict, low catering budget while maintaining high standards of nutrition. The media think this is a good story.

Draft a 200-word press release for a major national paper, and then a 400-word report for your internal newsletter. Think about the headlines you would expect to see in the tabloid press. What impact will this have on staff and patients?

The future of professional accountability

So what is the future of regulation for nursing?

The NMC Code of Professional Conduct is the main focus of regulatory accountability for nurses. All other professions have a different Code. There is likely to be growing argument to have a single Code of Conduct that applies across the UK to any health professional. There may be a detailed debate about whether all the regulatory bodies that govern health professions should be combined in a single body. There are likely to be moves to regulate health care assistants and other clinical staff who have a direct impact on patient care.

The voice of patients and clients is likely to be increased. The relationship between nurses and patients will become more open. There is likely to be a greater focus on the ways that nursing can develop to complement the needs of patients for access and information.

Quality health care will be measured and monitored by the regulatory bodies. These will work in different ways. Some will be UK-wide in their control, for example the Nursing and Midwifery Council. Others will be nationally based in their control, for example the regulators of social workers. The increased focus on devolution in health care will mean that different standards will be set by each UK country and this may lead to different standards being set for health professions in each country.

By now, you should be able to:

- understand the factors that influence professional accountability
- be confident about the role and function of regulation in professional accountability
- understand the key functions of the NMC
- describe the professional regulatory bodies that regulate individuals
- relate professional accountability across the range of health care settings
- assess what you think is needed to influence professional accountability.

Useful websites

Commission for Social Care Inspection: www.csci.org.uk
General Social Care Council: www.gscc.org.uk
Scottish Social Services Council: www.sssc.uk.com
Northern Ireland Social Care Council: www.niscc.info
Care Council for Wales: www.ccwales.org.uk
Council for Healthcare Regulatory Excellence: www.chre.org.uk
Nursing and Midwifery Council: www.nmc-uk.org

General Medical Council: www.gmc-uk.org
General Optical Council: www.optical.org
General Chiropractor Council: www.gcc-uk.org
General Dental Council: www.gdc-uk.org
Health Professions Council: www.hpc-uk.org
Royal Pharmaceutical Society of Great Britain: www.rpsgb.org.uk
General Osteopathy Council: www.osteopathy.org.uk
Royal College of Physicians: www.rcplondon.ac.uk
Royal College of Midwives: www.rcm.org.uk
Royal College of Nursing: www.rcn.org.uk
www.hmso.gov.uk/acts sets out legislation from Parliament.
Department of Health in England: www.dh.gov.uk
Welsh Assembly: www.wales.gov.uk/subihealth
Scottish Executive Health Department: www.show.scot.nhs.uk
Department of Health Social Services and Public Safety in Northern
    Ireland: www.dhsspsni.gov.uk
Financial Ombudsman Service: www.financial-ombudsman.org.uk

References

Council for Regulation of Health Care Professionals v. *Nursing and Midwifery Council
    and Steven Truscott* [2004] EWCA Civ 1356.
Department of Health (2002) *Code of Conduct for NHS Managers*, Department of
    Health, London.
Department of Health (2003) *Care Homes for Adults (18–65) and Supplementary
    Standards for Care Homes Accommodating Young People aged 16 and 17*, section
    25.4. National Minimum Standards, Care Homes Regulations. The
    Stationery Office, London.
General Medical Council (2001) *Good Medical Practice*, 3rd edition. GMC,
    London.
The Health Act 1999. The Stationery Office, London.
NHS Reform and Health Care Professions Act 2002. The Stationery Office,
    London.
NMC Order. *The Nursing and Midwifery Order 2001*. Statutory Instrument 2002
    No. 253, The Stationery Office, London.
Nursing and Midwifery Council (2002) *Code of Professional Conduct*. NMC,
    London.
Nursing and Midwifery Council (2004a) *Reporting Unfitness to Practise: a guide
    for employers and managers*. NMC, London.
Nursing and Midwifery Council (2004b) *Reporting Lack of Competence: a guide
    for employers and managers*. NMC, London.
Royal College of Physicians (2003) *The Vegetative State: guidance on the diag-
    nosis and management*. Report of a working party of the Royal College of
    Physicians. RCP, London.
Woolgar v. *Chief Constable of Sussex Police and UKCC* (1999) The Times, 28 May.

The Second Pillar of Accountability: Ethical Accountability

Learning objectives

Each nursing situation will involve individuals who have different health needs and different reactions to their wellbeing. Every person therefore has to be assessed individually. This raises many issues of ethical interest for nurses who consider the human dynamic of health but who may not understand some of the basic principles of ethical approaches to everyday dilemmas. This chapter considers some definitions and applications for a few key ethical values:

- autonomy
- paternalism
- utilitarianism
- equity
- best interests
- trust and truth
- acts and omissions.

The learning objectives for this chapter are to:

- understand the broad range of ethical issues that impact on nursing practice
- be clear about the basic ethical principles in nursing practice
- assess the relationship of ethics to health care
- assess the consequences for nursing practice of ethical accountability

Continued

- place ethical accountability in nursing in the framework of accountability
- be confident about the range of ethical issues in accountability.

Introduction

Societal values in nursing have changed over the years. The earliest cases involving misconduct by nurses in the 1920s tended to involve registered nurses being struck off after being found in hotel rooms with married men (Pyne, 1997). No cases of this sort have been heard by the UKCC or the NMC.

Personal values held by individual nurses are often subsumed by the need to be professional at all times as a nurse. This is a source of conflict for nurses who may have conscientious objections based on their personal beliefs about care, treatment, dignity or the behaviour of patients. Some nurses may have no difficulty in providing professional care to those who were convicted of child abuse or to women who want a pregnancy terminated, while others may struggle to provide care for such individuals. It depends on the particular set of values held personally by each nurse.

Ethics are the set of values based on a philosophical understanding that has been developed over thousands of years. The joy of a study of ethics in health care is that there is no single answer to any dilemma. It is radically different in that sense from a study of law in health care. However, there are systems of classifying ethical approaches that can be used in health care settings which remain constant, and which are applicable to nursing.

There are different systems to classify the main principles of ethics that apply in health care. One famous classification was created by the American philosophers Beauchamp and Childress which sets out four principles (Beauchamp and Childress, 2004). These are structured to allow a full discussion about ethical issues among those who have different views and different approaches to philosophy and healthcare ethics. These four principles are:

- respect for autonomy (respect the patient's choices)
- nonmalefience (do no harm)
- beneficience (do good)
- justice.

An understanding of key concepts in ethics can enable nurses to analyse and reason why any particular issue in their practice raises conflict, concern or a difference of opinion. It is a very valuable tool for justifying decision making in health care.

Summary

- Ethics cover the values that underpin the philosophy of nursing.
- A framework of ethics does not provide answers to complex problems.
- A framework can provide the basis for principled discussion.
- Different classifications include that created by Beauchamp and Childress.
- Societal values towards nursing have changed over the years.
- Personal values are important as part of a nurse's accountability.
- Nurses should be aware of their own values in nursing.

Activity

Consider what you believe to be the *worst* thing that:

- A nurse could do to a patient?
- A nurse could do to another nurse?
- A nurse could do to a member of the family of the patient?

What are your reasons for each answer?

Now consider what you believe to be the *best* thing that:

- A nurse could do to a patient?
- A nurse could do to another nurse?
- A nurse could do to a member of the family of the patient?

What are your reasons for each answer? Is there any relationship between your answers?

Autonomy

Autonomy is the value that society gives to each individual to choose what happens to his or her body, in the context of that individual's choices, preferences, values and lifestyle. It ensures that the person's right to determine what happens to his or her body is respected for matters including quality of life, peace of mind and self-respect. Autonomy allows an individual to make choices and have them treated with respect by others.

The intrinsic value of an individual is regarded as something so important to society that it has to be protected from external influence and undue coercion. Some moral philosophers such as Kant believed in autonomy as the highest societal value (Scruton, 2001). Respecting the autonomy of the patient is so important that it is often included in the Code of Conduct for health care professionals. It requires that others do not interfere with the decision making process of the individual even where the individual makes a decision that may increase their pain and suffering, or may shorten their life. This can be a hard value to uphold in nursing practice where the nurse is aware that there is some form of treatment that would lead to a more beneficial outcome in health terms for the individual.

Autonomy is given by society to those individuals who have the capacity to make these decisions for themselves. Where a person cannot exercise autonomy, the moral values used cover paternalism and best interests. Small children and those who are unconscious will not be able to exercise autonomy. Adults with mental impairment may have limited autonomy, depending on the nature of the impairment.

Public policy considerations are the principle used to ensure that the ethics of society are of greater importance than the rights of the individual. This will mean that limits are placed on the extent to which autonomy can be respected. Public policy can act as a brake on the ethical principles of autonomy and best interests by pronouncing that societal values are of a higher order. Most decisions about this balance are decided by the law, either through legislation or case law.

There may be situations where the ethics for the individual conflict with the ethics of society. Current debate centres around the extent to which resources can be limited even though this may conflict with the wishes and values of the individual.

In other cases a person may refuse all treatment including nursing care. Public policy may decide to respect the autonomy of the individual to a certain level, but place a limit on this autonomy. Public policy may require that an individual is not abandoned by society even where this is his autonomous wish.

Summary

- Autonomy is an ethical value that allows an individual to decide what happens to his or her body.
- Those choices may lead to the person choosing to refuse treatment.
- Codes of Conduct often reinforce the value of autonomy in health care.
- Autonomy may be a hard moral value for nurses to promote where they can see a more beneficial health outcome.
- Autonomy is given to those who can exercise this right.
- Public policy may place a limit on an individual's best interests.
- Public policy is where societal values are more important than the individual's values.
- Resources may be a key area where public policy decisions are made.
- Best interests are similar to autonomy and are used for those who lack autonomy.
- Public policy can restrict the extent to which best interests and autonomy are respected.
- Societal values can outweigh individual values.

Activity

The NMC Code of Professional Conduct places the autonomy of the patient very highly. Clause 2 states:

'**As a registered nurse, midwife or health visitor, you must respect the patient or client as an individual**

2.1 You must recognise and respect the role of patients and clients as partners in their care and the contribution they can make to it. This involves identifying their preferences regarding care and respecting these within the limits of professional practice, existing legislation, resources and the goals of the therapeutic relationship.

2.2 You are personally accountable for ensuring that you promote and protect the interests and dignity of patients and clients, irrespective of gender, age, race, ability, sexuality, economic status, lifestyle, culture and religious or political beliefs.

2.3 You must, at all times, maintain appropriate professional boundaries in the relationships you have with patients and clients. You must ensure that all aspects of the relationship focus exclusively upon the needs of the patient or client.

2.4 You must promote the interests of patients and clients. This includes helping individuals and groups gain access to health and social care, information and support relevant to their needs.

2.5 You must report to a relevant person or authority, at the earliest possible time, any conscientious objection that may be relevant to your professional practice. You must continue to provide care to the best of your ability until alternative arrangements are implemented.'

Read this clause through. Do you consider that it explains the importance of autonomy?

Paternalism

Paternalism in broad terms is where a person's exercise of autonomy is limited by another who wants to promote the welfare of that person. Every time a well-meaning parent tells a teenager to clean their room, take off that mascara or stop watching television, and every time a well-intentioned friend tells another to ditch a partner or to stop eating a doughnut, paternalism is affecting the autonomy of the individual.

Acting in a way that disregards the value of autonomy of the individual is paternalism. A nurse will want to promote the health of the individual to provide the best quality outcomes for the patient. A nurse has the expertise in different types of care and will use his or her judgement to assess which will provide the optimum outcome for patient. Over past decades, there was a strong sense of paternalism in the health service. Patients would queue up for instructions and follow the advice given without complaint. Nurses and doctors expected compliance with their advice. There was a shared understanding between the nurse and the patient that the nurse's advice and instructions were for the best.

The patient may disagree with the proposed action being set out by the nurse. This is where autonomy and paternalism conflict as values. The patient has disregarded the skill and judgement of the nurse without having the equivalent expertise to justify the decision. Some nurses will seek to persuade the patient to their way of thinking without realising that this compromises the fundamental right of autonomy. Other patients may agree with the logic of the course of action but just refuse for their own reasons to go ahead and have that treatment.

This is where paternalism can conflict with autonomy. Balancing the autonomy of the patient with the professional paternalism to provide the best health outcome is a complex aspect of ethics in nursing practice.

Summary

- Ignoring the individual autonomy of the patient is paternalism.
- The nurse and the patient may have different ideas about what is in the patient's best interests.
- Autonomy and paternalism may conflict with each other.
- Balancing autonomy with an instinct to be paternalistic is a challenge for nurses.

Activity

Patrick is a 17-year-old who has started taking heroin. His mother comes to the GP surgery because she wants to stop him taking this drug.

Discuss where you think the balance lies in the conflict between autonomy and paternalism in this case. Does the fact that heroin use may have a detrimental impact on those around Patrick at home make a difference to your discussion?

Utilitarianism

Utilitarianism is the moral principle that asserts there is no definite right or wrong in any action. The utilitarian approach is that any action is right or wrong only in relation to its consequence. That consequence must be to maximise happiness and minimise misery. In this way, a utilitarian approach to health care involves calculating the anticipated consequences of any situation and carrying out a risk assessment. This risk assessment will calculate the outcomes and then balance these to decide whether a greater good is achieved.

There are no set rules that have to be followed or set of values that are placed in an order of hierarchy. The course of action to be taken is the one that provides the greatest benefit at the least cost. The decision made is on the basis of doing the greatest good to the greatest number of people. The phrase 'the end justifies the means' is often used by those who follow a utilitarian approach.

The difficulty with utilitarianism is that it is hard to predict in advance the costs and benefits for any particular situation. Each situation has to be assessed at the time. People can be counted as a resource rather than as individually intrinsically valuable, and as a result there may be unease about calculating the value of an individual against the annual budget of running a clinic. However, this calculation is very often used in resource allocation where it is clear in advance that there will be insufficient resources to meet all the needs of the population.

Summary

- Utilitarianism is a moral calculation based on assessing how to obtain the greatest happiness and the least amount of misery.
- Resource allocation is often calculated on a utilitarian basis.
- This assesses the costs and benefits of treatment against the levels of need of the population.
- There are no set rules or hierarchies of values that are more or less important.
- No action is inherently right or wrong; it is the consequence that is measured.

Activity

Jamie is a very ill baby with significant intensive care needs. He is six months old and has already had five operations. The doctors decide that no further surgery would assist and that he only has a few months to live. The hospital may argue that the continued use of surgical interventions is not appropriate as it may mean that a disproportionate amount of resources are being requested that may only increase the life of the baby by a few months.

His parents disagree and believe that further intensive treatment will extend his life, even while they accept he may not survive. They argue that his intrinsic value as a child means that everything possible should be done to help

Continued

keep him alive. They do not accept that there should be a limit on the resources that are given to their child, and say that they have been paying into the NHS for years without needing major treatment.

Assess the arguments for the hospital and for the parents using autonomy and utilitarianism. How does an assessment of the moral issues help you define the arguments used by each side in this case?

Equity

Equity is a principle that requires distribution of resources, whether time, money or skills, based on achieving as close a balance as possible between members of society. A concern about equity was one of the main motivating forces behind the creation of the National Health Service. William Beveridge, the architect of the welfare state, argued for a health service which would provide treatment 'to every citizen without exception, without remuneration limit and without an economic barrier at any point to delay recourse to it' (Timmins, 2001). Equity has remained a major goal within the UK system.

Those that need greater resources are given them where this provides a way of bringing members of society into equity with each other. It is a way of measuring outcomes that give each individual equal value in society. In health care, it would mean that greater resources are given to those who are disabled or sick, at the expense of providing resources to improve the health of those who are already well.

Equity is different from utilitarianism in that it would allow greater resources to those who have greater need or greater disability, even where the outcomes may not be as cost effective as in a utilitarian approach. Equity allows a tolerance for individuals that may be disregarded by a utilitarian approach.

In health care, this approach to equity would mean that resources should be distributed according to need rather than according to the ability to pay. The debate then takes place about how best to define need, for example, emergency treatment to save life, or planned treatment to improve the quality of another person's life. Is it right to give expensive emergency treatment to a motorcyclist who crashed when he was travelling at 80 miles an hour because his needs are more urgent than those being provided through the chiropody services for older people? Need in this case may be defined as life-saving need, in which case those waiting for treatment that would improve the quality of care in their life but who are not in urgent need of treatment would wait until there were resources available to them. This would be justified on the principle of equity because those waiting for chiropody would be considered of lower priority based on a principle of need.

Summary

- Equity values each individual.
- It requires distribution of greater resources for those who have greater need.
- Utilitarianism and equity may conflict.
- Equity allows a tolerance and respect for individuals that may not be counted in utilitarianism.
- Utilitarianism is often used as a moral calculation in resource allocation.

Activity

Consider the arguments in resource allocation. A budget cut has to be adopted. The service most at risk is the community continence service. A meeting is held to assess the risks in cutting this service. The continence nurse is going to the meeting. She believes one of her strongest arguments is that the cuts should fall on the surgical department where significant resources are given to treating individuals who are obese or who have been smoking.

Sketch out the arguments you think she can use at this meeting based on the moral principles of equity. Assess what arguments you think she may face at the meeting from the staff in the surgical team.

Best interests

'Best interests' is the ethical principle used in decision making for those individuals who are unable to make their own decisions about their welfare. They lack the ability to be autonomous. These individuals may be babies, children who are unconscious, adults with a disability that affects their mental functioning or adults who have an early degenerative illness that means on some days they do have autonomy and on other days they do not. The principle of respecting the individual as intrinsically valuable is a key part of the principle of best interests.

Best interests cover the whole welfare, interests, values and known wishes of the person. It is now clear that best interests are not confined to *medical* best interests but must take into account the patient's values and preferences when competent, their wellbeing and quality of life, relationships with family or other carers, spiritual and religious welfare and their own financial interests. For very young children, the test of best interests has been applied by an assessment of the quality of life that is being considered.

Relatives do not have the final say on what the best interests of the individual should be, but their views should be respected. Sometimes there may be conflict among health professionals or family members over what the range of best interests covers, and in extreme cases where no agreement can be reached the case can go to court. In a hearing the court will decide what the best interests of the individual should be. Where the individual is a child, the child can be made a ward of court which means that the final decision making power over what would be in the child's best interests would be decided by the court, which carries out an independent assessment and determination.

One of the ways nurses can begin this discussion is to ask family and others close to the patient what they think the patient would want. Finding out values important to the patient is a way of obtaining information that will allow consideration of what option to take in the patient's best interests. This calls for sensitivity in dealing with family members who themselves may be in conflict over this.

Summary

- Best interests is the principle used for a person who cannot exercise autonomy.
- Best interests has a wider meaning than the best health interests.
- There may a conflict of views over what adds up to someone's best interests.
- The courts can decide what would be in a person's best interests.

Activity

Jeannette is a 29-year-old woman with severe learning difficulties. She has recently started a relationship with a man who visits her at home. Jeanette's mother approves of the relationship but is worried that if Jeanette becomes pregnant, she will be unable to deal with the pregnancy or with looking after the child. She suggests to the learning difficulties nurse, Tom, that a hysterectomy may be in Jeanette's best interests.

What issues would Tom need to consider in making his own assessment of the best interests of Jeanette?

Trust and truth

Truthfulness in the clinical relationship is an important part of nursing practice. It is important for the relationship because it reinforces the trust that is a necessary requirement in clinical practice. When a patient trusts that the nurse is acting in a way that maintains the dignity of this relationship, the reputation of the whole profession is enhanced.

This would suggest that it is important for a nurse to be honest in the clinical relationship. However, patients may not want to know their diagnosis or prognosis in some situations, particularly where this may be terminal. Brutal honesty may undermine respect of the dignity of the patient to receive information in a way and at a time that is appropriate for him or her.

Where a patient asks a direct question about proposed treatment, the nurse is under a moral duty not to lie. Telling the truth is fundamental to the basis of the relationship of trust between the nurse and the patient.

It is important that the nurse acts in such a way that she or he has the trust of the patient or client. Where this trust disappears there is a real prospect that the patient may withhold information because he or she no longer trusts what the nurse may do with it. This is a particular issue where the patient has information about their health that may be connected to some activity that is unlawful or distasteful to the nurse. It is important that the nurse is honest with the patient about the extent to which she or he will be dealing with that information. This is a way in which trust can be maintained between the nurse and the patient.

Some nurses may be concerned about the harmful effects of disclosing too much information to patients. Assuming that such disclosure is done with appropriate sensitivity and tact, there is little empirical evidence to support such a fear.

There are two main situations in which it may be justified to withhold the truth from a patient. If the nurse has compelling evidence that disclosure will cause real and predictable harm, truthful disclosure may be withheld, for example where disclosure would make a depressed patient actively suicidal. This withholding of the truth should only be used in situations when the harm seems very likely, rather than merely hypothetical. The second circumstance is if the patient asks not to be told the truth. Some patients might ask the nurse to talk to family members. In these cases it is critical that the patient gives thought to the implications of handing over their autonomy in decision making. If they made an informed decision not to be told, however, this preference should be respected.

Summary

- Trust is an important part of the nurse–patient relationship.
- Trust is the basis on which the patient can be honest with the nurse.
- Brutal honesty may not assist trust where this is inappropriate for the patient's dignity.
- The nurse has a moral duty not to lie when asked a direct question about clinical care.
- There may be situations where the risk of actual harm to the patient means the nurse wants to withhold the truth.
- In some situations, the patient may ask that the nurse gives information to family members only.

Activities

1. The NMC Code of Professional Conduct requires that nurses are trustworthy. Clause 7 states that 'As a registered nurse, midwife or health visitor, you must be trustworthy'. Clause 7.1 states that 'You must behave in a way that upholds the reputation of the professions. Behaviour that compromises this reputation may call your registration into question even if is not directly connected to your professional practice.'

   How far do you think this clause would allow a nurse to tell a patient information that was not truthful, as long as it meant there was still clinical trust in the relationship?

2. Niall is an intensive care nurse. He has been caring for Susan who was involved in a serious road traffic accident. Susan regains consciousness and calls for her husband. Niall knows that her husband was killed in the accident. He is concerned that if she knows this, she may slip back into a coma. He wants to reassure her so that she has a reason to maintain her recovery.

   Should he tell her the truth? How would this affect the trust in their clinical relationship if he did not tell her the truth?

Acts and omissions

The moral value of acts and omissions is important in end-of-life decision making, particularly by nurses. There is a moral difference between acts and omissions.

An act is defined as a positive action that is taken by the clinician. Where a patient is in pain and asks for pain relief, the decision to give morphine is an act.

An omission is defined as a positive decision to avoid taking an action. Where a child is near to death and is unconscious, an active decision not to intubate is an omission. Where a nurse sees an elderly patient in distress but chooses not to call the crash team, this is an omission.

The difficulty with the moral debate on acts and omissions is that the outcome for the individual patient may be the same, particularly at the end of life. Taking a positive action may be interpreted as an active engagement with the dying process of that person, and would be close to hastening the death of that person. This has been the subject of controversy over whether such an active engagement would be the equivalent of killing another person.

An example often used to highlight the moral dilemma in acts and omissions is whether it is morally worse to kill someone than to stand by and let them die. Is it worse to push someone into a river so that they die, than to come across a person in distress in the river and simply stand by taking no action? The first activity is an act, while the second activity is an omission.

The debate is that failing to intervene is an appropriate ethical response where the individual autonomy of an individual is concerned. There is no moral criticism for a person who did not come to the rescue of another in distress, because there is no moral imperative that demands intervention in another person's life. However, where an individual does act to cause the death of the other person, then that action can be criticised.

A further aspect to take into account in relation to acts and omissions is the doctrine of double effect. This doctrine has been developed largely in relation to death and dying. It is the doctrine that allows a primary action to be taken even though, as an unintended secondary consequence, the person may end up in a worse situation. The key example would be pain relief in a person who is dying. While it would be morally unacceptable to act in a way that hastens that person's death, it is accepted that the consequence of giving pain relief may hasten the death, even though that is not the prime reason for giving the drug. Where a prescription is given for pain relief, the primary purpose is to reduce suffering. As an unintended consequence of the prescription, the person may take such a large dose of the drug that he or she dies. Where the primary motive is pure, it outweighs an undesirable secondary effect.

Summary

- Acts and omissions are a complex moral topic generally focused on end-of-life issues.
- An act is a positive action taken by a clinician.
- An omission is a positive decision not to act.
- The outcome of the act or omission may be the same.
- There is greater moral criticism of someone taking an action than an omission.
- The doctrine of double effect allows a primary action to take place even though an unintended secondary action may also occur.

Activity

Heidi, a nurse practitioner, has given a repeat prescription to Sarah for her father who she is caring for at home. He is very ill. Sarah tells Heidi that she will inherit a large manor house in Dorset when her father dies and that she has been thinking of hiring an interior decorator to completely overhaul the

Continued

house. Heidi wonders whether Sarah will be influenced by the house in Dorset and whether she will decide not to give the medicine to her father so as not to prolong his life.

Consider the moral responsibility on Sarah in relation to acts and omissions if she decides not to give the medicine to her father.

Consider the moral responsibility on Heidi in relation to acts and omissions if she decides not to share her thoughts with anyone.

Application to accountability

The aim of this chapter has been to set out the broad range of ethical issues that have an impact on nursing practice. The importance of an understanding of the ethical issues is that the nurse can enrich an assessment of accountability by considering a range of moral issues for which there may be no concrete answer.

Many of the legal principles that apply to nursing practice will have a foundation in ethical issues. The prime moral principle upheld by the law is that of autonomy. Many legal decisions have criticised the use of paternalism on the part of clinicians where this may have affected or limited the autonomy of the individual. The NMC Code of Professional Conduct places a high value on the autonomy of the individual, considering it central to the maintenance of a professional relationship.

Employment practices may not be based directly on ethical principles, but in health care there will be many situations where the response of various individuals, whether the patient, family members or members of the health care team, differs. An understanding of the values that drive each of these individuals will enable the nurse to grow in compassion for the range of different views held.

By now, you should be able to:

- understand the broad range of ethical issues that impact on nursing practice
- understand the basic ethical principles in nursing practice
- place ethical accountability in the context of nursing practice.

Useful websites

Christian Medical Fellowship: www.cmf.org.uk
Bioethics Web: www.bioethicsweb.ac.uk
Ethics Research Information Catalogue: www.eric-on-line.co.uk/index.php
UK Clinical Ethics Network: www.ethics-network.org.uk
Bioethics and Society Research Register: www.bioethicsandsociety.org
Bioethics Today: www.bioethics-today.org

References

Beauchamp, T. and Childress, J. (2004) *Principles of Biomedical Ethics*, 5th edition. Oxford University Press Inc, USA.

Nursing and Midwifery Council (2002) *Code of Professional Conduct*. NMC, London.

Pyne, R. (1997) *Professional Discipline in Nursing, Midwifery and Health Visiting*. Blackwell Publishing, Oxford.

Scruton, R. (2001) *Kant: A Very Short Introduction*. Oxford Paperbacks, Oxford.

Timmins, N. (2001) *The Five Giants: A Biography of the Welfare State*. Harper Collins, London.

The Third Pillar of Accountability: Legal Accountability

Learning objectives

The legal context in nursing practice is an important part of accountability. The advantage of the legal process is that so much of it is defined. This means that nurses can always be clear what type of law applies to any clinical situation. In turn, this should lead to a greater sense of confidence among nurses about the law that applies to their practice.

This chapter aims to set out what law is, where it comes from, how it is made and who are the lawyers. In this way the overall objective is to show that the law at its heart has a logical structure that is capable of being influenced greatly by the voice of nursing. This chapter sets out the main structures of law so that it is placed firmly in the framework of accountability.

The learning objectives for this chapter are to:

- understand what the law is and why it is important
- understand the process of making law
- be able to identify different types of law and lawyers
- place law in the context of health care provision
- know where to turn to when the limits of the law need further explanation
- firmly place law in the framework of accountability
- clarify the key essentials of civil, criminal, public and European law.

Introduction

Many nurses report that they are not clear about the impact law has on their practice. This can lead to defensive nursing practice and unwillingness to place the needs of the patient above the potential risk of legal action. The legal principles in nursing may be poorly understood and therefore mistranslated among clinical staff. When cases go to court, they can attract great media interest. Cases that go to court will always have a human interest element and a debate that has not been resolved between the parties.

This can be a frustration to judges who have been keen to ensure that, when complex health issues reach the courts for a hearing, a nursing voice is heard to counterbalance arguments between managers, doctors, patients or their family members. The reality is that most of the health law cases heard in courts focus on medical decisions. Hardly any cases focus on nursing decisions. At the same time, an increasing number of nurses are now training to be lawyers as their interest in health care is influenced by an interest and enthusiasm for the legal framework in health care.

In the broadest sense it is possible to say that the law is based on practical common sense. As a result, the principles that underpin the law in health care are easy to understand. The application to specific areas of practice is where the limits of this framework are tested.

As the number of court cases in health care increases, the relevance of an understanding of law to nursing practice becomes more important. Where nurses are confident about the application of law to their practice, this will provide a greater clarity in the nurse–patient relationship.

Summary

- A poor understanding of law can lead to defensive nursing practice.
- Cases that are heard in court can attract significant media interest.
- Most court cases focus on medical decisions rather than nursing decisions.
- There are an increasing number of health care cases being heard in court.
- More nurses are becoming interested in law.
- In a broad sense, law is based on practical common sense.
- An understanding of law leads to confident nursing practice.

Activity

Look at the UK legislation website at www.hmso.gov.uk/acts/acts1992.htm. Which Acts of Parliament that year have an immediate health connection? Of all the Acts shown for that year, which one surprised you most and why?

What is law?

Law is the system by which a society agrees that various rules and penalties are used to provide a common framework by which each member of society lives. Law is a series of rules, and interpretations of those rules, that have to be followed by citizens of a country. The law can set penalties if the legal rules are broken. The legal process provides a structure for the law to be made and refined, for disputes to be resolved and how individuals can be represented in those disputes.

The law in the UK covers every aspect of life, including health care. The European Union is another source of law that must be followed in each country of the UK.

In broad terms, the law comes from both *legislation* and from *court cases*. Different courts and tribunals hear disputes about the interpretation of legislation, and where their decisions are followed by other parties in similar disputes, this creates a *precedent*. The law made in interpreting legislation or earlier court cases is called *case law*.

Summary

- Law is a set of rules and penalties agreed by society.
- Legal disputes are resolved in different courts and tribunals.
- Law covers every aspect of life, including health care.
- Law is made through legislation and by court cases.
- Court cases provide case law.
- Where case law is used in other cases, it becomes precedent law.

Activity

What Act of Parliament would you want to introduce on any subject? What would you want to contain, control, forbid or encourage by this Act? Can you think of anyone who would be unfairly affected by this Act? How long do you think it would take to turn this idea into legislation?

Why is law important?

Law represents the rules that reflect the values of a society at any stage in its history. Where society alters its value structure, the law has to reflect this. For example, the punishment for murder used to be death by hanging. This was changed in the second part of the twentieth century as society decided that hanging was no longer a preferred option. The penalty now is life imprisonment. There is still a strong sense in society that murder is the most serious criminal activity, so the longest sentence is regarded as appropriate.

Parliament is made up of Members of Parliament who are elected by the people of a particular constituency. These politicians decide the law that is to be made in each parliamentary session. The political party that has the overall majority in Parliament will set out the law for the following year in the Queen's Speech each November. The Acts of Parliament passed therefore reflect the political aims of the party with the greatest majority in the House of Commons at the time.

In criminal law, society regards it important to have a representative section to decide whether an individual is guilty or innocent. In the magistrates' courts this will be done by magistrates and in the crown court it will be done by a jury. The jury is made up of individuals who are called to serve as a cross-section of society. Everyone who is on the electoral register is able to be called for jury service.

Summary

- Law represents the values of a society at any given time.
- Values can change over time and the law changes with this.
- MPs reflect the values of their constituents in Parliament.
- Parliament makes laws that reflect these values.
- Criminal law has an input from a representative sample of society.

Case study 4.1: Legislation challenge

Diane Blood was faced with two situations where the wording in Acts of Parliament prevented her from acting in a way that felt appropriate to her circumstances. The wording in the Human Fertilisation and Embryology Act 1990 prevented her from using frozen sperm from her husband who had tragically died from meningitis. The Act requires the donor's consent in writing for the sperm to be used. This was clearly not possible as Mr Blood had died. Diane Blood was able to take the frozen sperm to Belgium where the law did not have the same requirements for written consent. She continued with her fertility treatment and gave birth to a son.

Diane Blood lobbied for the Act to be changed. She argued that the circumstances that affected her were not considered at the time the Bill was making its way through Parliament. The Government set up a review of the legislation but has not changed the Act.

She then discovered a second problem with the wording in the Human Fertilisation and Embryology Act 1990 when she was told that she could not have her late husband registered as the father of her child. As a result of her lobbying activities she persuaded enough politicians that a change was needed, and the Act was amended by the Human Fertilisation and Embryology (Deceased Fathers) Act 2003.

Continued

This shows two things. First, the way that Acts of Parliament are worded may lead to unintended consequences for people. Secondly, where an Act of Parliament sets boundaries that do not work in practice, it is possible to use the courts to challenge the interpretation of the wording. In some cases the law can be changed after sustained lobbying of Parliament.

R v. *Human Fertilisation and Embryology Authority ex parte Blood* (1997)

Where is law made?

Legislation is law that is passed by Parliament. It covers the whole population and sets out in precise language what people, agencies or the Government must do. It will also set out what agencies or the Government may do. Legislation also sets out the penalties when the prohibited activity takes place. Where an activity takes place that is specifically not allowed by legislation, this is *unlawful*. Where the legislation has put penalties in place if this action takes place, this is *criminal*. Nothing can be regarded in law as criminal unless it is contained in legislation.

Legislation covers Acts of Parliament (primary legislation) and Statutory Instruments (secondary legislation). Legislation sets out the functions, duties and penalties for many aspects of an individual's life. It also sets out the functions and powers of agencies created by the Government, such as the Nursing and Midwifery Council (NMC). If the NMC attempts to act in a way which goes beyond the powers set out in its legislation, the person affected by the action can ask the court to review that action and if necessary make a decision that it was unlawful. This type of challenge to legislation is known as a *judicial review*.

Members of Parliament are involved in deciding how to scrutinise the legislation that is being passed through Parliament by the Government of the day.

Case law is created by judges in courts that cover either civil law or criminal law. The judges will interpret disputes over the meaning of words or intentions in legislation so that there is a clear understanding of the rules that apply. In criminal cases, the judge will be assisted by a jury which decides whether a person is guilty or not.

Figure 4.1 shows the court structure in England and Wales for civil, criminal and public law cases.

Summary

• Legislation is law that is passed by Parliament.
• Legislation will set out what actions are prohibited and actions that must be taken.

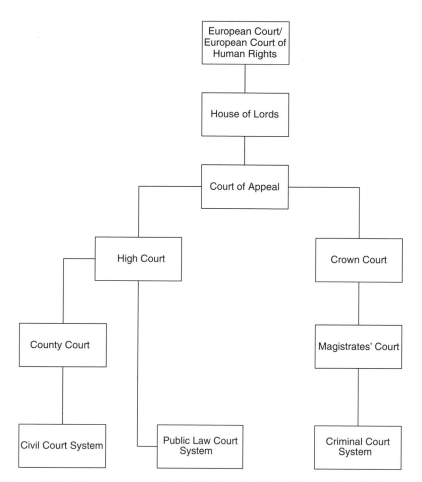

Figure 4.1 Court structure in England and Wales for civil, criminal and public law cases.

- It will set out penalties where prohibited actions take place.
- Legislation covers Acts of Parliament and Statutory Instruments.
- Judicial review is a challenge to the actions of a public agency.
- Parliament passes legislation through its MPs.
- Courts decide on disputes between individuals in civil law.
- Courts decide whether an individual has contravened legislation, with a jury involved in criminal law.
- Courts also decide how legislation is interpreted.

How is law made?

An Act of Parliament can only be changed by another Act of Parliament. Once the Act of Parliament has been passed, Parliament can make secondary legislation known as Statutory Instruments. Secondary legislation is approved by Parliament but is much quicker to make into law than an Act of Parliament. As a result, it can be amended more easily. There is a structured process for making legislation. An Act of Parliament is made in the following way:

- A Green paper is published which sets out why the Government thinks an Act of Parliament is needed. This is the consultation stage, where the public and organisations can send in responses suggesting ways that this problem can be addressed in legislation or by giving examples of how there may be unintended consequences of the proposals that need to be considered.
- A White paper is published setting out the way the Government will take matters forward.
- A Bill is published in either the House of Commons or the House of Lords.
- The Bill has a first reading where the title is read out and a statement is made about the intent of the Bill.
- The Bill has a second reading where the principles are debated in broad terms by MPs or Lords.
- The Bill goes to Committee where amendments can be considered and accepted or rejected.
- The Bill goes back to the House of Commons for report stage where a general discussion takes place on the amendments.
- The final Bill is then voted on by both the House of Commons and the House of Lords.
- If the Bill is passed it becomes an Act of Parliament.
- The Queen signs the Act of Parliament with the Royal Seal.
- The Act of Parliament is now law.

Criminal law is where an individual breaks a requirement in the legislation. In criminal cases the state will fund the prosecution case, but may ask the defendant to pay costs towards the case if the defendant is found guilty.

Civil law is made by judges. The judge will hear both sides of the case that is put forward by lawyers. Witnesses may be called to give evidence either about what they saw at the time or as expert witnesses to give an informed opinion on matters that are outside the general knowledge of the lawyers.

In civil cases the general rule is that the loser of the case pays his own costs as well as the costs of the winner of the case. For this reason there have to be strong arguments to take a civil case to a hearing because of the costs risk involved. Where the individual does not have the means to pay for the case, it is possible in some circumstances to apply for legal aid. This means that the state pays for the cost of the case. There are also some centres that provide *pro bono* advice, where lawyers provide legal skills for free.

In both criminal and civil law cases, the decision made by the court can be challenged by the losing party, generally if they feel that there was an improper use of the legal process or that the judge made some error of law. The appeal is to the higher court in the system, and in civil law cases as each appeal is heard there are more judges who sit in the court:

- High Court   1 judge
- Court of Appeal   3 judges
- House of Lords   5 judges

Each judge will give a written judgement and, from this, new clarification about aspects of the legal issue under discussion will be made. In general, the courts have to follow the legal principles that have been set by earlier courts. This is known as following precedent.

Summary

- Legislation has a structured process for its creation.
- Criminal law hears cases where an individual has broken an Act of Parliament.
- Case law is made by judges who follow a precedent set in other cases.
- Paying for the court case is a reason that deters individuals taking civil cases.
- Appeals in both criminal and civil cases go to a higher court.
- Precedent is set by following rules set down in earlier cases.

Activity

Who is your Member of Parliament? You can find out by looking at the website www.parliament.uk. Read his or her biography. Do they have an interest in health care in your constituency? If there is an area that you do not feel is being covered, write a letter to your MP saying why you think it is important they take an interest in this area.

Case study 4.2: Amending an Act of Parliament for nursing activity

The thorny issue of nurse prescribing has arisen largely as a result of legislation. The Medicines Act 1967 provided in section 57 (2) (b) the specific identities of the professionals who could supply prescription only medicine, restricted to doctors, dentists and vets. Because the clause was so specific, it

Continued

meant there was no prospect of nurses having legislative authority to supply prescription only medicine.

Because an Act of Parliament can only be amended by another Act of Parliament, it was not until the passing of the Medicinal Products: Prescription by Nurses etc. Act 1992 that nurses had the power to prescribe. This Act altered section 57 in the earlier Act so that other 'classes' of persons, who were not defined in professional groups in the 1968 Act, could be allowed to supply prescription only medicines if they had complied with specific education, training or professional requirements.

This paved the way for nurses to have the legal ability to supply medicines and then become nurse prescribers.

Who are lawyers?

'Lawyers' is the general word given to all those who are qualified in some way to practise law. Lawyers in England and Wales can only practise in England and Wales, lawyers in Scotland can only practise in Scotland and lawyers in Northern Ireland can only practise in Northern Ireland.

Paralegals

Paralegals are not qualified lawyers but may have some academic background or experience in law. An increasing number of nurses work in solicitors' offices and are employed as paralegals.

Legal executives

Legal executives generally work in solicitors' offices. They obtain their qualifications through the Institute of Legal Executives (ILEX). They are less qualified than solicitors. There are limits on the extent to which they are allowed to appear in court.

Solicitors

Solicitors advise clients on any aspect of law. Most solicitors choose to specialise in a particular area of law, and there are now fewer generalist solicitors than in the past. Some may cover mental health or family law, while others may work on property or commercial law. Where the solicitor needs to access specialist skills in legal research or advocacy, the solicitor will instruct a barrister to carry out a particular piece of research or advocacy in court. Solicitors must have a practising certificate that is renewed each year by the Law Society, and must maintain three-yearly continuing professional development. Each UK country has a Law Society that regulates solicitors.

Barristers

Barristers are self-employed lawyers and specialise in legal research, advice on complex issues or advocacy. Barristers in England and Wales are trained at one of five Inns in London following which they are called to the Bar. The Bar Council keeps a register of barristers and is the regulatory body for barristers in England and Wales. Barristers cannot yet advise clients directly although this rule is about to change. At present, the barrister relies on being chosen by a solicitor to appear in court on behalf of the client. When a barrister has been practising for 10 years, he or she can apply to become a recognised Queen's Counsel (QC).

Judges

Judges tend to be barristers by background. They sit in court and listen to the arguments being put by both sides in the case. Judges have to be impartial. They have to make sure that the correct legal process is followed in a case. In criminal cases, the judge will tell the jury the process they have to follow when deciding whether the facts of the case can lead to a finding of guilty or not guilty. In civil cases there is no jury so the judge will be the person who decides the outcome of the case.

Law Lords

Law Lords are judges who consider cases that are on appeal. They decide whether the law made in the lower courts was correct. If they do, the appeal will be dismissed. If they find the law was not correctly interpreted, they will uphold the appeal.

Activity

Look at the Law Society website or the Bar Council website for your country (these are set out in the websites at the end of this chapter). See if you can find a solicitor or barrister in your area who specialises in health law. Do they offer lectures or newsletters by which you can update yourself on health law developments?

Types of law

The types of law that can be heard in courts are:

- civil law, which involves disputes between individuals
- criminal law, which involves disputes between the state and the individual
- public law, which involves the relationship between the citizen and the state

- European law, which involves the relationship between the rights of EU citizens and EU states.

Civil law

Civil law covers all areas of law that involve a dispute with a private element in the relationship. Civil law covers the following by way of example:

- family law
- disputes between neighbours
- wills
- conveyancing and the transfer of property
- nuisance
- employers' liability for accidents
- employment law
- negligence
- consent
- confidentiality.

One of the real problems with civil law is that it can only be developed if the right case comes to court at the right time. Even where nurses think there may be a gap in the way their nursing practice could be clarified by the courts, they generally have to wait for an individual to experience that situation and decide to ask the court to decide the outcome. Taking a case to court costs money and the outcome can never be guaranteed. To make matters worse, the general rule is that if you lose a case, not only do you pay your own legal costs but also the legal costs of the other side.

Summary

- Civil law covers relationships that have a private element to the relationship.
- Cases in civil law only go to court when an individual decides to argue their case.
- It is never possible to predict the outcome of a court case in civil law.
- The cost of taking a case to court means that fewer cases are heard than may exist.
- Nurses can take cases to court where they feel there is a conflict in their nursing practice.

Case study 4.3: Giving expert evidence

An expert in a court case has a crucial role to play. He or she will write a report setting out the facts of the case, and will then reach written conclusions about whether and how the outcome of the incident could have been avoided. If the case is not settled, it may go to court. The expert will give evidence in court based on the content of the report and answer questions put by the barristers in court relating to the way in which those conclusions have been reached, or expanding on the technical information contained in the report.

Cross-examination by the other party's solicitor is the part of the expert's job which many dread. Cross-examination involves the other party's barrister trying to undermine the content of the report in an effort to discredit the standing of the expert or the content of the report. In that situation it is necessary for the expert to answer as accurately as possible, even if the expert knows that the answer will not help the client's case.

The common approach for barristers cross-examining a witness is to find an inconsistency in the report. Experts generally cope with this by listening to the questions very carefully and answering them accurately. If an expert does not know the answer to a question, he or she should say so.

Giving evidence in court is a nerve-racking experience. There is no easy way around this. Once you are in the witness box giving your evidence as an expert there will be no one for you to turn to for assistance. It is vital that the content of your written report is something that you are completely confident about.

It is important to remember that the expert is there to assist the court to establish what happened, when and why. The expert does this by giving factual evidence of the incident or treatment which is in dispute. It is not for the expert to take sides in the litigation. The expert is independent and objective about the particular expertise they are commenting on.

Always listen carefully to the question. Think before answering, answer only the question asked and be concise. Never try to argue with the barrister putting the question to you. Remember that barristers are experts themselves in arguing. Do not be drawn away from your field of expertise. If you are a nurse with expertise in lifting and handling of patients, you may not be able to answer questions on aspects of, say, community nursing which are not directly connected with lifting and handling. Do not try to become an expert in aspects where you have no knowledge. If you restrict yourself to the particular expertise you have, your own reputation will be enhanced.

Criminal law

Criminal law is concerned with the rights between the state and the individual. All criminal cases that go to court are in the name of the Queen as head of state, to show that criminal law is a matter of society enforcing rules on an individual.

Types of criminal activity range from serious crime such as rape or murder through to lesser crimes such as traffic offences. One feature that marks criminal law as different from civil law is that a finding of guilt in criminal law usually results in some form of punishment. This is to show that society does not want that type of behaviour and will use punishment as a deterrent against that behaviour. The punishment can be custodial, when a prison sentence is made, or non-custodial, when a sentence of community service or a fine is made.

Criminal law is an important part of nursing practice because it is set out in Acts of Parliament. If one person steals property from another the legislation used in the criminal case is the Theft Act 1968, which at section 1(1) says 'a person is guilty of theft if he dishonestly appropriates property belonging to another with the intention of permanently depriving the other of it'. If a community nurse making home visits takes a DVD from a patient without permission the nurse is acting unprofessionally, but if the nurse intends to return it on her next visit she has not committed a criminal offence.

All criminal cases are first heard in magistrates' courts in front of magistrates. The magistrates' courts can hear straightforward cases. Where a case is more complex or the sentence that may be given is longer than the magistrates have the power to give, the case will be referred to the crown court. Where cases are heard in crown courts, there will be a jury to decide whether the evidence proves that the legislation has been infringed beyond reasonable doubt. If a person is found guilty, the judge will decide the penalty to be imposed.

Summary

- Criminal law is the relationship between the state and the individual.
- Criminal law sets out the boundaries of behaviour required by the state.
- All crown court cases are in the name of the Queen as head of state.
- Criminal law is followed by punishment when a finding of guilt is made.
- Punishment can be custodial or non-custodial.

Activity

Find the local magistrates' court and go there for a morning to listen. Tell the clerk that you are watching to see how law is made. Watch the way the magistrates find out the facts. Would you have asked other questions?

Public law

Public law is a mechanism by which an individual can challenge the powers that are given to the state or to agencies of the state. Where a civil servant misinterprets guidance, and the outcome is that an individual is deprived of their rights, the courts will hear the case under public law. This is sometimes called administrative law because it is about the way the administration of the state, public authorities and office holders carry out their functions.

Areas of public law include:

- education
- health care
- immigration
- welfare benefits
- retirement pensions
- pollution
- community care
- housing
- social work
- compensation for victims of crime.

Where an individual believes that he or she has been wrongly or unfairly treated by the rules that apply to any of these areas, it is possible to apply to the court for a judicial review. This is a request that a judge reviews the decision or the policy under which the dispute arises. One of the most influential areas in recent years in public law is community care law, particularly around the funding of continuing care.

An issue decided by judicial review will have an impact on the rest of society or at least a section of society that is in a similar position to the individual.

Summary

- Public law is heard in court using a process called judicial review.
- The outcome of the case will apply directly to the individual but will impact on a section of society.
- Public law is concerned with the way the state makes decisions about an individual.

Case study 4.4: Public law challenge: Long-term care funding

Pamela Coughlan challenged the basis on which she was being means tested for the nursing care being given to her in a care home. She argued that because she had multiple difficulties arising from a road traffic accident, all her nursing care should be funded by the NHS.

She took a judicial review to the Court of Appeal, against the decision of the North and East Devon Health Authority. The case was so significant that both the Secretary of State and the Royal College of Nursing appeared in the Court of Appeal to argue wider issues of the definition of nursing and its funding.

The Court of Appeal found that where the reason for being accommodated in a care home was primarily for health care, then the whole of the care home treatment and costs should be funded by the NHS.

R v. North and East Devon Health Authority ex parte Coughlan (2000)

European law and devolution in the UK

The impact of European law on the way that law is made in the UK is significant. The UK has agreed to follow the rules and laws of the European Union. This means that citizens of the UK can have a right to apply to the courts in Europe if they feel that decisions made by the courts in the UK are not compatible with the wider laws of Europe.

One of the most important parts of European law is the European Convention on Human Rights, which is now part of UK law. Many health care cases that are taken to the European Court of Human Rights are based on a conflict of interpretation of the Convention. Chapter 7 sets out more detail on human rights.

Acts of Parliament made in England will generally also apply to Wales. As the impact of devolution takes place, it is likely that Wales will start to develop its own Statutory Instruments for the implementation of rules that are particular to Wales in health law. Devolution in Scotland means that in health law, Acts of Parliament for Scotland are now made by the Scottish Parliament. Legislation in Northern Ireland in health law is intended to come from the Northern Ireland Assembly. Where there are different Acts of Parliament and different Statutory Instruments, there will be different challenges made in the courts about the applicability and interpretation of this law. The courts in each UK country will take account of what has been said in the courts of another country, but they are not under an obligation to follow law that does not apply in their country.

Summary

- European law has a significant impact on UK law.
- UK citizens can apply to European Courts if they are not satisfied with the UK court ruling.
- The European Convention on Human Rights has had a significant impact on health care law in the UK.
- Devolution in the UK means that greater differences in the legal systems of each UK country are likely.

Activity

Find out who is your European Member of Parliament by looking on the website at www.europarl.org.uk. See if they have a surgery near you. Go along and ask what they are doing for health care across Europe.

Case Study 4.5: European law and assisted suicide

Dianne Pretty achieved major media interest sympathetic to her case. She suffered from motor neurone disease. She did not want artificial ventilation but was anxious not to die by choking. She wanted her husband Brian to assist her to die when she felt that her disability became unbearable.

This was a problem in law because the provisions of the Suicide Act 1961 state that assisting another person to die is a criminal offence. She applied to the court for a declaration that if her husband did carry out this action he would not be prosecuted for manslaughter.

Dianne asked the House of Lords to consider that this Act was incompatible with the European Convention on Human Rights. The House of Lords did not agree that there was a conflict. The House of Lords had to read and interpret the provisions of the Suicide Act. They decided that the proposed action by Diane's husband would be a criminal activity under the legislation.

Dianne Pretty went to the European Court of Human Rights in March 2002, and died in May 2002. The European Court of Human Rights held that the provisions in the Suicide Act 1961 were justified as a protection for adults who were dying and vulnerable.

Pretty v. *UK* (2002)

Application to accountability

The law is a significant aspect of accountability for nurses. It can create the most anxiety in nursing practice where the limits on legal accountability are not clear. Chapters 8 and 9 set out the key concepts in law that most closely affect nursing practice in negligence and consent. Chapters 10 and 11 show how the sources of law affect specific areas of nursing practice in confidentiality, conscientious objection and palliative care.

Where nurses want to assess their legal accountability, they should first check whether there is legislation that covers the particular area. If not, they should check what previous case law may exist. This will be the key approach that any lawyer would take in deciding whether an answer to the issue raised has already been dealt with.

Where a new point of law arises in nursing practice, it is important to assess whether this can be taken to court for a resolution. To do so may mean that other nurses who face a similar situation will gain legal guidance about how best to continue with their nursing practice.

By now, you should be able to:

- identify the sources of law
- explain how an Act of Parliament is made

- avoid defensive nursing practice
- assess what engagement you can have in the development of case law
- be confident about the relationship between law and nursing.

Useful websites

www.hmso.gov.uk/acts is a key site that has a full copy of all Acts of Parliament and Statutory Instruments from the Westminster Parliament.

Law Society for England and Wales: www.lawsociety.org.uk
Law Society for Scotland: www.lawscot.org.uk
Law Society for Northern Ireland: www.lawsoc-ni.org
Institute of Legal Executives: www.ilex.org.uk
Bar Council for England and Wales: www.barcouncil.org.uk
Faculty of Advocates (Scottish Bar): www.advocates.org.uk
Bar Council for Northern Ireland: www.barcouncil-ni.org

www.bondsolon.com offers training in expert witness report writing and giving evidence in court.

References

European Convention for the Protection of Human Rights and Fundamental Freedoms (1950), Council of Europe, Strasbourg.
Human Fertilisation and Embryology Act 1990. The Stationery Office, London.
Human Fertilisation and Embryology (Deceased Fathers) Act 2003. The Stationery Office, London.
Medicinal Products: Prescription by Nurses etc. Act 1992. The Stationery Office, London.
Medicines Act 1967. The Stationery Office, London.
Pretty v. *UK* [2002] 2 FCR 97.
R v. *Human Fertilisation and Embryology Authority ex parte Blood* [1997] 2 All ER 687.
R v. *North and East Devon Health Authority ex parte Coughlan* [2000] 3 All ER 850.
Suicide Act 1961. The Stationery Office, London.
Theft Act 1968. The Stationery Office, London.

The Fourth Pillar of Accountability: Employment Accountability

Learning objectives

The relationship between an employer and an employee brings the fourth and final pillar of accountability into focus. With an increasing number of nurses choosing to work independently, either as agency, bank or self-employed, it is important to understand the relationship of employment in the framework of accountability. This chapter will set out a brief description of the types of employment relationship, the rights and protections that apply in each type of employment relationship, and the role of protocols and policies.

The learning objectives for this chapter are to:

- understand the different types of employment relationship
- be clear about the key elements in a contract of employment
- apply the use of protocols and policies to the employment relationship
- consider basic employment rights of:
  - discrimination
  - family rights
  - unfair dismissal
  - redundancy
- realise the impact of the Working Time Directive
- place the role of employment in any nursing situation in the framework of accountability
- be confident about the place of employment in the framework of accountability.

Introduction

Where an employment relationship exists, a number of rights are given to the nurse such as her or his entitlement to time off for maternity or paternity leave, as well as protection against different types of discrimination in the workplace.

There are now different types of employment relationship as nurses move away from the 'job for life' approach to their career. Other rights are relevant to nurses in different types of employment relationships, such as bank nurses, agency nurses or self-employed nurses.

Where a nurse is employed on a full-time basis, she or he will have a contract of employment which will set out the duties and responsibilities for the nurse. There may be other protocols or policies that the employer expects of the nurse and these may be set out in supporting documents.

Where an employment relationship breaks down, employment tribunals can be used to obtain remedies for the rights that may exist, such as unfair dismissal or redundancy payments.

An understanding of how employment practice fits within the framework of nursing accountability will help nurses become more confident about the application of the employment relationship in their practice.

Summary

- Nurses in different employment relationships may be full-time employed, part-time employed, bank, agency, apprentices or self-employed.
- Different employment relationships provide protection against discrimination.
- Contracts of employment set out rights and responsibilities for the nurse.
- Policies and protocols provide further structure in the employment relationship.
- Different employment relationships provide rights of protection for maternity and paternity leave.
- Different employment relationships provide rights of protection against unfair dismissal or redundancy.
- Employment tribunals hear cases for unfair dismissal and redundancy claims.

The employment relationship

The employment relationship is largely defined in the Employment Rights Act 1996, the main legislation. Chapter 4 sets out how legisla-

Table 5.1 Tests to decide whether a person is an employee.

Name of test	Which assesses
Control test	Whether the client paying for the services has control over the individual
Organisation test	Whether the person's contribution is essential to the business rather than being an accessory to it
Economic reality test	Whether a person is working for himself or working for another
Multiple test	How much reliance is placed on the person's own work and skill in the business arrangement
Mutuality of obligations test	The obligations owed by each of the parties to each other, particularly useful in cases involving casual workers and homeworkers.

tion is made. One of the key ways to show that an employment relationship exists is to have a contract of employment (Employment Rights Act 1996, section 230 (1)). Where this does not exist, other factual evidence can be used. The courts have developed a system of 'tests' to decide whether a person is an employee for the purposes of applying for legal rights. Table 5.1 sets out these tests.

A European Directive (EC 91/533) has dealt with the employment relationship, and questions to ask when deciding whether a person is an employee include:

- date the relationship began
- how long it is expected to last
- normal working time
- remuneration.

Issues to be resolved arising from a dispute between the employer and the employee are generally heard in employment tribunals. The employment tribunal has a legally qualified chairman who sits with two other members drawn from business and employment. An appeal can be heard in the employment appeal tribunal, with further appeals to the Court of Appeal and the House of Lords. Employment tribunals hear cases that deal with:

- unfair dismissal
- redundancy payments
- discrimination
- contract claims.

To bring a claim against an employer, the employee fills in form ET1 with the nature of the grievance and the remedy being looked for. The remedy may include reinstatement or compensation if the person is claiming rights of unfair dismissal or compensation if the person is claiming redundancy. A person who is not in an employment relationship which carries these rights cannot claim these rights. The Advisory, Conciliation and Arbitration Service (ACAS) has a Code of Practice on Disciplinary and Grievance Procedures (ACAS, 2004) that recommends what should be in a disciplinary process and how mediation can be used to avoid hearings at an employment tribunal.

Summary

- A series of tests has been devised in the UK and in Europe to discover whether someone is an employee so the rights that go with that relationship can be claimed.
- Different employment rights are given to those who can show they are in an employment relationship.
- Cases involving a dispute are heard in an employment tribunal.
- ACAS provides mediation services to assist cases before they reach an employment tribunal.

Case study 5.1: Duty to provide honest references

In a case heard in 1984, the court found that a duty of care could arise in negligence on the part of the employer in giving a reference.

Where the former employer says that the individual is trustworthy, even though he knows that the individual has a history of petty theft, any new employer would be able to claim that the reference was negligent and sue for compensation if they discovered that the new member of staff had stolen property.

It also works the other way. Where a former employer gives a poor reference that is used as a reason not to give someone a new job, this reference can be challenged on grounds of negligence if the content was incorrect.

Spring v. *Guardian Assurance PLC* (1994)

Activity

Look at the Employment Tribunal website www.employmenttribunals.gov and find out if there is a hearing centre near you. Find a day when you can sit in and see what claims are being made. Were you surprised at how informal it was, or do you think that suited the nature of the case?

Types of employment relationship

Full time

Full-time workers on a permanent contract have access to the fullest range of employment rights. The limits on these rights may depend on the length of time that the person has been in full-time employment with the same employer. For example, rights to remedies for unfair dismissal apply to those in full-time employment after one year; rights to payment for redundancy apply after two years' employment.

Part-time

Part-time workers have special protection which gives them the right not to be less favourably treated than full time workers (Part-time Workers (Prevention of Less Favourable Treatment) Regulations 2000). Part-time workers have a proportionate equivalent of benefits such as salary, sick pay, maternity pay and occupational pension schemes given to full-time counterparts.

Activity

Sally works part-time in a job share with Sandra. Sally works Wednesday to Friday and notices that she misses out on Bank Holidays which fall on Mondays. Calculate how many Bank Holidays fall in each year, and decide how you would suggest Sally takes this up with both Sandra and her employer.

Fixed-term

The individual is employed on a fixed-term contract for a specific amount of time, or for a specific piece of work, or for a specific event. They have protection under the Fixed-term Employees (Prevention of Less Favourable Treatment) Regulations 2002. This is similar to the protection for those who are part-time. From 10 July 2002, if a person has been employed on successive fixed-term contracts for four years or more, then the next time that contract is renewed it will be regarded as a legally permanent contract.

Trainees

A contract of apprenticeship is regarded as a contract of employment (Employment Rights Act 1996, section 230 (2)), so trainees with a contract of apprenticeship are protected by employment rights. Not all trainees are apprentices and those who do not have this contract have no contract of employment. Nursing students need to be clear whether they have a contract of apprenticeship which would provide this protection. Even if this is not the case, they do have protection in equal opportunities and in health and safety.

Agency

Nurses who obtain work through an agency are self-employed and have very limited employment rights. The client will have a contract with the agency and will pay the agency an agreed amount that will include the nurse's services and the agency's fee. The key legislation is the Employment Agencies Act 1973, with further details in the Conduct of Employment Agencies and Employment Businesses Regulations 2003. This provides, for example, that the agency must carry out background checks on individuals before offering their services.

Bank

A nurse can apply to be on a list of those available to work for an NHS facility. This is known as being on the bank. There is no guarantee of work. There is no contract of employment, even though payment for working a shift on the bank may be paid through the payroll of the NHS facility. Bank status is the overtime basis for staff in the NHS. There is also an NHS Code of Practice for the Supply of Temporary Staffing that sets out requirements to ensure that nurses and other health care staff who work in this way are provided with continuing professional development (Department of Health, 2002). In a case in 1998, a bank nurse was denied a global contract of employment as the Health Authority argued that it could not guarantee her any work. She was simply able to work as and when needed. The question of whether she had a contract of employment each time she worked was sent to the employment tribunal who assessed this based on the tests shown in Table 5.1 (*Clark* v. *Oxfordshire Health Authority* (1998).

Self-employed

A person who is self-employed is not in an employment relationship, unless he or she becomes an employer by taking on staff. Where the self-employed person provides products or services to another organisation or to an individual, it is for the self-employed person to organise the payment of fees, deductions for tax and National Insurance, and where necessary to become VAT registered.

Summary

- There are different types of employment relationship.
- A nurse may have several different employment relationships at one time.
- Different protections and rights affect each type of employment relationship.

The contract of employment

The contract of employment can be agreed orally or in writing. It is much easier to see the terms of the contract of employment if they are written and signed by both parties. All employees are entitled to a written statement of initial employment particulars no later than two months after the beginning of employment (sections 1–7 of Employment Rights Act 1996). This must contain:

- names of the employers and employee
- date on which the employment began
- date on which the employee's period of continuous employment began
- rate of pay
- intervals at which the pay is made (weekly, monthly)
- terms and conditions relating to hours of work
- terms and conditions relating to holiday pay, sick pay, pensions
- length of notice on either side
- job title or a brief job description
- whether the employment is permanent or fixed term
- the place of work or where various locations are situated
- collective agreements that affect the terms and conditions
- whether the employee is expected to work outside the UK
- any disciplinary rules and procedures applicable to the employee.

The employer has duties to:

- pay wages
- indemnify the employee against liabilities and losses incurred during the course of employment
- provide work
- take reasonable care of health and safety
- take reasonable care in giving references.

The employee has duties to:

- obey orders and instructions from the employer
- exercise reasonable care and skill in carrying out the contract of employment
- exercise good faith in carrying out the contract
- not disclose confidential information.

Other wider rights may apply to all workers through legislation. For example, the National Minimum Wage Act 1998 provides that all workers, whether agency, home-workers or part-time, must not be paid below a certain level decided by the Low Pay Commission. Exclusions to this right apply to those aged under 18 and to those on an apprenticeship contract.

Summary

- A contract of employment can be written or agreed verbally.
- There are specific matters that must be included in a statement of employment.
- There are legal duties placed on employers and employees.
- Other wider rights apply to all workers, such as the right to a minimum wage.

Activity

Look at your contract of employment. What terms and conditions do you expect to see there? How would you redraft this to reflect your current employment?

Protocols and policies

Most health employers will have a set of protocols and policies that are intended to provide elaboration of the main provisions of the contract of employment. These may cover specific areas of practice relating to health and safety, such as the range of warning signs that need to be placed in an area when cleaning is taking place. They may include details of how to carry out a particular nursing activity, such as ear syringing. In many cases, nurses are directly engaged in developing and refining protocols and policies that are used in the workplace.

The impact of these protocols and policies is that they form part of the employment relationship between the nurse and the employer. They may be used as part of any disciplinary process where an issue arises about whether the content of the protocol was followed correctly.

It can be tempting to create a protocol that gives a full account of best practice to be followed in any nursing procedure. There are two points to bear in mind: every protocol and policy should be dated, and should have a fixed date for further review. This will enable all staff to see at a glance whether the particular protocol is still effective. The second point is the need to distinguish what *must* be included in the protocol. This will cover the basic steps that cannot be ignored and has to be separated from what *may* be included in the protocol – which will cover those further aspects of nursing practice that achieve best practice but which are not critical to the safe performance of the task.

Summary

- Protocols and policies extend the employment relationship.
- Nurses may be directly involved in drafting policies and protocols.
- Every protocol and policy should be dated with a review date.
- It is important to clarify what *must* be done from what *may* be done.

Working Time Directive

The Working Time Directive was adopted by Europe in 1993. It was incorporated into UK law in the Working Time Regulations 1998.

It provides that no one should work more than an average of 48 hours a week measured over 17 weeks. This means that a nurse can work long shifts with overtime for several months, as long as over 17 weeks she can measure that she does not work more than an average of 48 hours a week.

Night shift is treated slightly differently. Normal night hours must not exceed an average of 8 hours for each 24 hours, measured over 17 weeks. This can be altered by collective agreement between the employer and one or more trade unions. Certain categories of workers are excluded from the regulations, including those who work in the armed services, the police and civil protection services. Doctors in training used to be exempted but this ended in 2003, and as a result doctors are now treated like every other health worker.

Summary

- The Working Time Directive has applied to nurses since 1998.
- It became effective for doctors in training in 2003.
- Junior doctor hours were reduced steadily between 1998 and 2003.
- Average numbers of hours worked are calculated differently between day shifts and night shifts.

Discrimination

Discrimination may occur where a person from a particular group claims that he or she has not been treated in an equal way with another person. For example, a GP surgery which wants to employ a nurse to set up a smear clinic may advertise for a female nurse. A male nurse would be able to bring a claim on the grounds of sexual discrimination. Even if the motive is well intentioned, there may be discrimination. Discrimination may be direct where treatment is less favourable because of generalised assumptions about the class of people involved. It may be indirect discrimination where the action would cause adverse impact to a considerably larger group or where it would disadvantage particular groups of workers.

The law provides protection against discrimination for part-time and fixed term employees. Sources of law that prohibit discrimination are from European Directives which have been adopted into UK law, as well as from the European Convention on Human Rights. Table 5.2 sets out the UK and European sources that prohibit different types of discrimination.

Table 5.2   UK and European sources that prohibit different types of discrimination.

Type of discrimination	UK law	European law
Sex discrimination	Sex Discrimination Acts 1975 and 1986 Sex Discrimination (Indirect Discrimination and Burden of Proof) Regulations 2001	Directive on Equal Treatment (76/207)
Sexual Orientation	Employment Equality (Sexual Orientation) Regulations 2003	Framework Directive (2000/78)
Transsexuals	The Gender Recognition Act (2004)	
Sexual harassment	Sex Discrimination Act 1975	Equal Treatment Directive 2000
Pregnancy	Sex Discrimination Act 1975	Pregnant Workers Directive 92/85
Race	Race Relations Act 1976 Race Relations Amendment Act 2000 Race Relations Act 1976 (Amendment) Regulations 2003	Race Discrimination Directive (2000/43)
Disability	Disability Discrimination Act 1995 Disability Rights Commission Act 1999	Framework Directive (2000/78)
Age	Regulations are to be made by 2006	Framework (Equal Treatment) Directive (2000/78)
Religious belief	Employment Equality (Religion and Belief) Regulations 2003	Framework (Equal Treatment) Directive (2000/78)
Equal pay	Equal Pay Act 1970	Equal Pay Directive 75/117
Equal treatment		Equal Treatment Directive 76/207

A complaint against discrimination must generally be made within three months of the event, except for a claim under equal pay which must be made within six months.

The remedies are those that can be claimed by the individual:

- compensation
- an order declaring the rights of the individual
- a recommendation that specific action is taken by the employer to reduce the discrimination
- an order that the employer makes reasonable adjustment for those with disability.

The Government has created some agencies with a remit to provide an overview of how different types of discrimination can be avoided. These agencies include the Equal Opportunities Commission, the Disability Rights Commission and the Council for Racial Equality, all of which have functions to:

- conduct investigations
- take action against discriminatory advertisements
- seek injunctions to restrain persistent cases of discrimination
- provide information and advice
- promote equal opportunities.

Summary

- There are different types of discrimination.
- European law has set out ways in which each can be identified.
- UK law has set out remedies for anyone claiming discrimination.

Family rights

The rights to time off work and rights to pay for family reasons are complex. This section sets out a broad structure of where these rights exist. The entitlement to these rights may depend on the amount of time that the individual has been employed.

There are different types of family rights:

- time off for antenatal care
- not to be dismissed because of pregnancy
- maternity pay and leave
- paternity pay and leave
- parental leave.

A pregnant woman has a right to take time off for antenatal care. There is no minimum length of service that the woman needs to have worked to be entitled to this right.

Dismissal because of pregnancy is not allowed, under the EC Pregnant Workers Directive (92/85). This provides protection against dismissal in any of the following circumstances:

- while pregnant or for any reason connected with it such as miscarriage
- during maternity leave
- because the woman took maternity leave
- suspension while on maternity leave
- redundancy while on maternity leave.

Where a woman is dismissed for any of the grounds above, she can claim that this was unfair dismissal.

Maternity leave, covered by the Maternity and Parental Leave Regulations 1999, provides two types of maternity leave: ordinary and additional.

Ordinary maternity leave provides a woman with a right to 26 weeks' maternity leave which can begin at any time from the 11th week before the expected week of the birth. This is a right of all employees no matter how long they have been employed. All other employment benefits that would have existed if the woman were not on maternity leave still apply, such as annual leave. The woman has the right to return to her previous job on the same terms as before. Failure to allow a woman to return counts as automatic unfair dismissal.

Statutory maternity pay is paid by the employer for these 26 weeks, for the first 6 weeks at 90% of the individual's average pay and then at a flat rate for the other 20 weeks, which at the time of writing is £106.00 per week. Many employers choose to pay more than this rate.

Additional maternity leave can last a maximum of 26 weeks after the end of ordinary maternity leave, giving a total of one year's maternity leave. This right is only available to women who have completed at least 26 weeks' continuous employment by the end of the 15th week before the expected week of childbirth. There is no statutory maternity pay for additional maternity leave.

On her return to work after maternity leave, a woman is entitled to the same job or another suitable and appropriate job.

Paternity leave and pay will give fathers two weeks' paid leave following the birth of their child as long as the father has 26 weeks' continuous employment. Statutory paternity pay, at the time of writing, is £106.00 per week or 90% of average earnings, whichever is the lower.

One member of a couple who adopt a child can take ordinary adoption leave (26 weeks' paid leave) and additional adoption leave (26 weeks' unpaid leave). The rights match those of maternity leave. Their partner may be entitled to paternity leave and pay.

Parental leave applies during the first five years of the child's life or until the 18th birthday of a disabled child. A maximum of 13 weeks is given for each parent but there is no right to be paid for this leave. Those who adopt children can take this leave during the first five years of the placement. One year's continuous employment is required for this right.

Time off to care for dependants gives a right to all employees to take time off to provide assistance when a dependant is ill or injured. A dependant is defined as wife, husband, child, parent or someone who lives with the employee.

Summary

- Family rights are given protection in the employment relationship.
- Family rights relate to protection against dismissal.
- Family rights give time off work for both men and women for the birth of a child and during the child's early years.
- Family rights apply for those adopting and for providing care to dependants.

Unfair dismissal and redundancy

Unfair dismissal can be claimed after one year's employment. This may take place where the employer sacks a person and the person claims this was unfair. The main reason for dismissal on the part of the employer will be based on the conduct of the employee. The claim for unfair dismissal on the part of the employee will be that the dismissal took place and that the employer acted unreasonably in treating the reason as sufficient for dismissal.

The case will be heard by an employment tribunal which will decide whether the reason for dismissal was reasonable. There are five potentially fair reasons for dismissal:

- lack of capability or qualifications of the employee
- conduct of the employee
- redundancy
- a legal statutory provision would be broken if the employee continued to be employed
- some other substantial reason that justifies dismissal.

Claims must be made within three months of the effective date of termination of the contract. Remedies for unfair dismissal are:

- compensation
- re-engagement
- reinstatement.

Redundancy occurs where a job will no longer exist (i.e. is redundant), so the employee doing it is no longer required and is dismissed. The employee is entitled to redundancy pay if they have been employed by the same employer for two years or more. It is possible to argue that no redundancy exists if an offer of suitable alternative employment is made. If the employee refuses this offer it may mean that the employee loses any right to a redundancy payment.

Where a person moves from one employer to another, if both employers are regarded as associated employers it may be possible to add the time worked for the first employer to the continuous employment for the second.

Summary

- Unfair dismissal and redundancy are both forms of dismissal by an employer.
- Unfair dismissal can be claimed after one year's employment.
- An employee is entitled to redundancy pay after two years' employment.
- There are rules to decide whether unfair dismissal or redundancy has taken place.

Case study 5.2: Redundancy

Under section 146 (1) of the Employment Rights Act 1996 an offer of alternative suitable employment may be made by an associated employer. If a nurse is being made redundant from an independent healthcare provider, but is offered suitable alternative employment by another independent healthcare provider that is counted as an associated employer, she may lose her rights to a redundancy payment if she refuses this offer.

An associated employer means that one of the companies has direct or indirect control of the other, or a third party has direct or indirect control of both companies (section 231, Employment Rights Act 1996). Case law has shown that the provisions relating to redundancy or unfair dismissal only apply if at least one of the employers is a company. Case law has also shown that the provisions relating to associated employers in the case of redundancy (or unfair dismissal) do not apply if the employers are public bodies, including Health Authorities. In *Gardiner* v. *Merton London Borough Council* a man who had worked for four local authorities would not be able to claim unfair dismissal unless he had worked for more than a year with one of them, but could add together all the time to claim continuous employment for redundancy purposes. This may apply where the nurse works in the private sector.

Gardiner v. *Merton London Borough Council* (1980)

Case study 5.3: Continuous employment and unfair dismissal

Sally started work in outpatients for West Charles NHS Hospital Trust on 1 January 2005. She left on 1 July 2005, and moved with her family to North Aspen NHS Trust. She had only worked there for a further six months before she was dismissed for lack of competence on 1 January 2006. She wants to claim unfair dismissal.

She only has six months' employment with the North Aspen NHS Trust, but if she can add the time she worked with the West Charles NHS Hospital Trust, she can show that she has a year's continuous service. As a result she would be able to begin a claim for unfair dismissal. If all the employment cannot be counted as continuous service, she cannot consider a claim of unfair dismissal as she has not achieved the minimum time limit.

Health and safety

Health and safety is an important aspect of employment accountability. There is always the option to sue an employer in negligence where the actions or omissions of the employer lead to injury. There is also a statutory framework for health and safety in the Health and Safety at Work Etc. Act 1974. Where an employer is found to have broken some aspect of the legislation, it will face a fine imposed by the Health and Safety Commission. There is also the prospect of criminal sanctions in certain circumstances.

Main duties from the Act include, in section 2(1), that 'it shall be the duty of every employer to ensure, as far as reasonably practicable, the health, safety, and welfare at work of all his employees'.

Section 2(2) sets out the areas in which the employer has to provide safe systems:

- the provision and maintenance of plant and systems of work that are safe and without risks to health
- arrangements for ensuring safety and absence of risks to health in connection with the use, handling, storage and transport of articles and substances
- the provision of such information, instruction, training and supervision as is necessary to ensure the health and safety at work of employees
- as regards any place of work under the employer's control, the maintenance of it in a condition that is safe and without risks to health, and the provision and maintenance of means of access to and egress from it that are safe and without such risks
- the provision and maintenance of a working environment that is safe, without risks to health, and adequate as regards facilities and arrangements for welfare at work.

The Health and Safety Commission is responsible to the Secretary of State for Work and Pensions. The Commission's functions are:

- to secure the health, safety and welfare of persons at work
- to protect the public generally against risks to health or safety arising out of work activities and to control the keeping and use of explosives, highly flammable and other dangerous substances
- to conduct and sponsor research, promote training and provide an information and advisory service

- to review the adequacy of health and safety legislation and make proposals to the Government for new or revised regulations and approved codes of practice.

The Health and Safety Executive is responsible for enforcing the Act and giving guidance to employers. Inspectors, who are employed by the Executive, have the following legal powers:

- to issue an improvement notice where the inspector believes that a provision of the Act is being broken
- to issue a prohibition notice where the inspector believes that activities are about to involve the risk of serious personal injury. The activity has to stop until the remedy is put in place
- to take articles or objects that the inspector believes may threaten imminent danger of serious personal injury.

Safety Committees and Safety Representatives are appointed by trade unions where these are recognised by the employer. There is a right to time off work with pay to perform these duties (SRSCR, 1977). They can:

- inspect premises
- investigate accidents and complaints from employees
- consult inspectors
- receive information.

The European Union has produced a 'six pack' of Directives that deal with aspects of health and safety. These Directives have been incorporated into UK law by the use of regulations:

- Management of Health and Safety at Work Regulations 1992
- Workplace (Health, Safety and Welfare) Regulations 1992
- Provision and Use of Work Equipment Regulations 1992
- Personal Protective Equipment Regulations 1992
- Health and Safety (Display Screen Equipment) Regulations 1992
- Manual Handling Regulations 1992.

Application to accountability

The employment relationship can be complex. Employment is an important part in the framework of accountability, particularly in nursing as the vast majority of nurses are in one or more employment relationships. The employment relationship affects the rights and duties that exist between the nurse and her employer, and has an impact on how she or he will deliver nursing care. An understanding of the employment relationship will enable nurses to assess what rights in employment exist, and the duties that arise on both the employer and the nurse as a result.

Protocols and policies are flexible and can shape the development of the contractual relationship. The rights of the employee are protected in legislation, much of which has its roots in European Directives. This demonstrates the fundamental importance of providing a structure of protection for the workforce.

Links to the other pillars in accountability will mean that in every nursing situation a review of the impact of professional, legal and ethical accountability can be mapped against the employment setting, so that the implications of any situation can be roundly considered.

By now, you should be able to:

- understand the different types of employment in nursing accountability
- realise the responsibilities and limits in a contract of employment
- assess the value of protocols and policies in employment
- set out the legislation for different types of discrimination in employment.

Summary

- Employment relationships can be complex between the nurse and the employer.
- Employment is about the rights and duties in the employment relationship.
- Rights and duties are protected, particularly by European Directives.
- Links across the four pillars of accountability will enable the nurse to make a rounded assessment of any nursing situation.

Useful websites

The Department of Trade and Industry has a useful website on the Working Time Directive at www.dti.gov.uk/er
Employment Tribunals: www.employmenttribunals.gov.uk
Employment Appeals: www.employmentappeals.gov.uk
Low Pay Commission: www.lowpay.gov.uk
Advisory, Conciliation and Arbitration Service: www.acas.org.uk
Equal Opportunities Commission: www.eoc.org.uk
Disability Rights Commission: www.drc-gb.org
Commission for Racial Equality: www.cre.gov.uk
Health and Safety Commission and Health and Safety Executive: www.hse.gov.uk

References

Advisory, Conciliation and Arbitration Service (2004) Code of Practice on Disciplinary and Grievance Procedures, ACAS, London.
Clark v. Oxfordshire Health Authority [1998] IRLR 125.
Conduct of Employment Agencies and Employment Businesses Regulations 2003 (SI 2003/3319). The Stationery Office, London.

Department of Health (2002) *NHS Code of Practice for the Supply of Temporary Staffing*. Department of Health, London.

Disability Discrimination Act 1995. The Stationery Office, London.

Disability Rights Commission Act 1999. The Stationery Office, London.

EC Pregnant Workers Directive (92/85).

EC Terms and Conditions of Employment Directive (91/533).

EC Working Time Directive (93/104).

Employment Agencies Act 1973. The Stationery Office, London.

Employment Equality (Religion and Belief) Regulations 2003. The Stationery Office, London.

Employment Equality (Sexual Orientation) Regulations. The Stationery Office, London.

Employment Rights Act 1996. The Stationery Office, London.

Equal Pay Act 1970. The Stationery Office, London.

Fixed-term Employees (Prevention of Less Favourable Treatment) Regulations 2002 (SI 2002/2034). The Stationery Office, London.

Gardiner v. *Merton London Borough Council* (1980) 1RLR 472

Gender Recognition Act 2004. The Stationery Office, London.

Health and Safety at Work Etc. Act 1974. The Stationery Office, London.

Health and Safety (Display Screen Equipment) Regulations 1992. The Stationery Office, London.

Management of Health and Safety at Work Regulations 1992. The Stationery Office, London.

Manual Handling Regulations 1992. The Stationery Office, London.

Maternity and Parental Leave Regulations 1999 (SI 1999/3312). The Stationery Office, London.

National Minimum Wage Act 1998. The Stationery Office, London.

Part-time Workers (Prevention of Less Favourable Treatment) Regulations 2000 (SI 2000/1551). The Stationery Office, London.

Personal Protective Equipment Regulations 1992. The Stationery Office, London.

Provision and Use of Work Equipment Regulations 1992. The Stationery Office, London.

Race Relations Act 1976. The Stationery Office, London.

Race Relations Act 1976 (Amendment) Regulations 2003. The Stationery Office, London.

Race Relations Amendment Act 2000. The Stationery Office, London.

Sex Discrimination Act 1975. The Stationery Office, London.

Sex Discrimination (Indirect Discrimination and Burden of Proof) Regulations 2001. The Stationery Office, London.

Spring v. *Guardian Assurance PLC* [1995] 2 AC 296.

SRSCR (1997) Safety Representatives and Safety Committee Regulations 1977 (SI 1977/500). The Stationery Office, London.

Working Time Regulations 1998 (SI 1998/1833). The Stationery Office, London.

Workplace (Health, Safety and Welfare) Regulations 1992. The Stationery Office, London.

Structures: The Health Service

Learning objectives

This chapter sets out the main components of a health service and the quality functions of the key agencies in England. This will enable nurses to place the NHS in context with the independent and private sectors in relation to rights and resources in accessing treatment and care.

The learning objectives for this chapter are to:

- fully describe the key components of any health service
- understand where the UK provides rights to access treatment and care
- assess the different sources of funding available for treatment and care
- review the quality standards in a health service
- place this in the context of agencies in England that assess quality of treatment and care.

Introduction

The National Health Service (NHS) is funded by taxpayers to provide a comprehensive service of health to all citizens of the UK. The independent sector is funded privately and provides services that may match or complement those provided in the NHS. Further health services may be provided by organisations that are voluntary or commercial, non-profit making or profit making.

The policy of universal coverage of health care from the NHS provides:

- primary care
- secondary care
- continuing care
- social care
- public health.

The Health Service and devolution in the UK

The health service is now devolved among the four countries of the United Kingdom. Since 1997 devolution across the UK has meant that England, Wales, Scotland and Northern Ireland can make health policy for their own country. This health policy is limited in different ways in each country, but overall the intention is to provide each country with responsibility for deciding its own health policy and how this is to be provided. Each Government will decide its priorities in health and then use the civil service to implement that health policy. Policy making for the structures of the NHS is carried out by a central government department in each UK country.

Devolution in health means that each country has some power to make its own decisions in relation to health:

- Parliament in Westminster can make primary legislation that may cover all or any part of the UK.
- Scotland can make its own legislation and can increase taxation for the population if it wants to raise income for health.
- Wales has an Assembly that cannot make its own primary legislation but can make its own secondary legislation.
- Primary legislation for England is dealt with by Parliament in Westminster.
- Northern Ireland has an Assembly (suspended at the time of writing), similar to the Assembly in Wales in that it can pass its own secondary legislation while the primary legislation is made by Parliament in Westminster.

Summary

- The NHS was set up to provide universal coverage of health for UK citizens.
- The health service is made up of services that provide primary, secondary, continuing care, social care and public health.
- The health service is devolved across the UK.
- Scotland makes its own legislation and can raise taxes for the NHS.
- Wales cannot make its own primary legislation but can make secondary legislation.
- Northern Ireland cannot make its own primary legislation but can make secondary legislation.
- Legislation for England is dealt with by Parliament in Westminster.

Activity

Go to the relevant health department website for the country that you live in. These are all listed at the end of this chapter. Have a look to see what changes and news are being presented on the first page. Then compare this with the website of any one of the other three country health departments. Look at the main differences in presentation of information. Make a bookmark note of your own health department website so that you can visit this on a regular basis to keep up with current changes.

Primary care

Primary care is the overall description of health services that are provided as a first point of call for the patient. Primary care services cover GPs, general medical services, pharmacists, dentists and opticians.

The services that exist in a geographical location are decided by the local NHS structure which will provide funding for the service in each country:

England   Primary Care Trusts
Scotland   Community Health Partnerships
Wales   Local Health Boards
Northern Ireland   Local Health and Social Care Groups

Technology means that increasing information is available via the internet or by call centres. NHS Direct is a nurse-led system that provides phone advice to anyone regardless of their geographical location. Databases mean that nurses can take a call and run through protocols to provide advice to those who call. Nurses at NHS Direct can arrange to send an emergency ambulance where needed. NHS Direct has a website where a range of information about different conditions is given.

Summary

- Primary care covers care provided by GPs, dentists, pharmacists and opticians.
- Primary Care Trusts in England fund primary care services.
- Technology means that primary care can be provided by nurses at NHS Direct.
- The NHS Direct website encourages people to look up information themselves.

Activity

Look at the NHS Direct website at www.nhsdirect.nhs.uk for the advice given on care of diabetes. Are you satisfied with the information that is set out? Critically evaluate whether you would want different information to be provided.

Secondary care

Secondary care is the care that requires more intensive health services and broadly covers surgical investigation, hospital stay and accident and emergency services. Access to hospital services is arranged by the GP who acts as gatekeeper to decide which service is most appropriate. The exception to this is accident and emergency services at major hospitals which are accessible by anyone needing emergency treatment.

A broader range of secondary services is being developed, with a focus on nurse-led services such as minor injury units to provide immediate care for less intensive forms of accident and emergency treatment.

Secondary services are provided in each country by:

England	Acute NHS Trusts
Scotland	NHS Trusts (Acute and University Trusts)
Wales	NHS Trusts
Northern Ireland	Health and Social Services Trusts

Access to ambulance services can be requested by anyone, although the NHS will now charge for the use of ambulance services by those who are later able to recover compensation for their injuries. Ambulance services are provided by:

England	Ambulance Trusts
Scotland	Special Health Board of Scottish Executive
Wales	Welsh Ambulance Services NHS Trusts
Northern Ireland	Northern Ireland Ambulance Service Trust

Summary

- Secondary care covers ambulance and hospital services.
- Hospital services are generally accessible through a GP.
- Accident and emergency services are accessible by anyone.
- Ambulance services can be called upon by anyone but claims for a refund may be made in some circumstances.

Continuing care and social care

Continuing care is provided for individuals on a long-term basis. This may cover those who have long-term conditions such as multiple sclerosis or those whose overall health is so vulnerable that they are unable to continue living an independent life without assistance on a continuous basis. Systems of continuing care can be provided in the individual's own home, where the services are provided by the state. Where the vulnerability of the individual becomes greater, for example, the risk of falls is greatly increased for a frail widow living alone, continuing care can be provided in a licensed care home.

Continuing care services are provided by:

England	Primary Care and Acute NHS Trusts
Scotland	Primary Care Trusts (Community Care Partnerships)
Wales	NHS Trusts and Local Health Boards
Northern Ireland	Health and Social Services Trusts

Social services are provided by local authorities. These are services that are not directly related to health care. Social care is the interface between health and social care where the social aspects of an individual may mean that, while health needs are important, they are secondary to the social care needs of that individual.

Social care services are provided by:

England	Local Authorities
Scotland	Scottish Executive Health Department and Local Authorities
Wales	Local Authorities and Local Health Boards
Northern Ireland	Health and Social Services Trusts

Summary

- Continuing care is provided on a long-term basis.
- It can be provided in the person's own home or in a care home.
- Care homes may provide residential care or nursing care.
- Social services are not directly related to health care.
- Social care is the interface between health and social services needs.
- Social care is provided where the social care needs are more important than the health needs.

Public health

Public health covers the range of services designed to promote the health of the population rather than the health of an individual. Public health services cover programmes to remove the causes of ill health and to prevent disease.

Research in public health will consider the mortality patterns of the population. This measures the death rate and may investigate changes in patterns relating to age, gender or employment background. Other research may focus on morbidity, which measures the incidence of ill health. This may consider the effect of lifestyle changes on the prevalence of asthma or eczema, for example. Other research may consider:

- sanitation
- clean air
- disease prevalence
- environmental factors such as pollution
- income factors and stress

- genetic factors
- diet.

Public health services may involve setting up vaccination services for widespread diseases such as polio or mumps. They may also involve services designed to assist the individual for the greater good of society, such as the focus on giving up smoking.

Public health services are provided by:

England	Health Protection Agency/Chief Medical Officer
Scotland	NHS Health Scotland/Chief Medical Officer
Wales	National Public Health Service for Wales/Health Protection Agency/Chief Medical Officer
Northern Ireland	Health Promotion Agency/Chief Medical Officer

Summary

- Public health can focus on the community rather than the individual.
- Public health research can measure mortality and morbidity rates.
- Individual services in public health can contribute to the greater good of the community.

Rights to treatment and resources

Sources of rights to treatment and resources

There is no set of principles set out in legislation for the NHS. This has been considered over the years, most recently in the *NHS Plan* (Department of Health, 2000) which stated that the NHS should:

- be comprehensive
- give equality of access to health care
- be equitable, with equal service for equal need
- be free at the point of delivery.

The NHS was created by an Act of Parliament. The most recent major NHS Act was passed in 1977. Section 1 of this Act sets out the prime duty on the Secretary of State for Health to 'promote a comprehensive health service' that will improve the physical and mental health of the population and will improve the prevention, diagnosis and treatment of illness. The legislation also provides that these services must be funded by general taxation and that no charges can be made to the individual receiving the service unless other legislation makes this a specific charge.

It is important to be aware that there are statutory duties for the Secretary of State in relation to the NHS. These duties give the Secretary of State the prime responsibility in relation to provision, funding and accessibility of a range of services. Where an individual wants to challenge the limitations on any treatment available in their area, the main source of the rights will be in the NHS Act 1977.

The legislation is crucial in deciding the source of the right to treatment and resources. Where the legislation states that the right to treatment or resources exists, the individual has the legal right to challenge any attempt by a health provider to deny access to these treatments or resources.

The legislation also sets out the basis on which some services can be charged for, and other services which must be funded centrally. Charges can be made to cover costs that arise after road traffic accidents where a negligence claim is successful under the Road Traffic (NHS Charges) Act 1999. Charges can also be made for optical and dental care, and for drugs. Charges can be made for those who are not resident in the country, except in an emergency. When deciding whether a health service is funded by general taxation or whether a charge can be made to the individual, the starting point is whether there is any legislation.

Case law has considered whether the rights set out in the legislation have been properly understood by the Secretary of State over the years. These cases involve the courts looking at the policy that has been decided, measuring this against the rights to treatment and resources that are set out in the legislation, and then deciding whether there is a match between the two. If there is not, the courts will order that the Secretary of State alters the policy.

Summary

- Legislation will be the source for deciding what treatment is available on the NHS.
- The basic principle is that the Secretary of State has a duty to promote a comprehensive health service.
- This is not the same as a universal right to any treatment or resource.
- Charges cannot be made for NHS services except where allowed by legislation.

Case study 6.1: Assessing the limits on policy provision

A young girl known as B was 10 years old when diagnosed with leukaemia. Both her specialist consultant in Cambridge and specialists at the Royal Marsden Hospital treated the child with bone marrow transplants but decided that further treatment was inappropriate. She was given a prognosis of only a few months. Her father consulted other doctors including a professor at

Continued

Hammersmith Hospital who discussed a new form of experimental treatment that was being carried out in America involving a new form of chemotherapy. This was being assessed to find out whether patients may be well enough to undergo a further bone marrow transplant. The Cambridge Health Authority refused to fund this experimental treatment on two grounds: that it was not clinically supported treatment and that it would use disproportionate resources.

The father took the case to court and argued that the treatment would be in his daughter's best interests. The court found that the treating medical specialists were better placed to decide what was in the best interests of B, and that it was not for the court to overrule this clinical assessment. The court considered the issue of resource allocation and decided that while the NHS Act 1977 gave obligations to the Secretary of State, it was for each Health Authority to make its own decisions about resource allocation.

R v. *Cambridge Health Authority ex parte B* (1995)

Sources of funding

Funding of the health service is provided by general taxation. There are different systems of funding primary care, secondary care and continuing care that are set out in the NHS Act 1977 and subsequent NHS Acts that specifically focus on the structures of each aspect of health service provision.

The independent sector provides health care that is funded directly by the individual. There is no central system of funding for the provision of independent sector care, although where the NHS needs to expand its capacity, it may negotiate a contract with an independent sector provider to create additional surgery or post-operative treatment. This may mean that the patient has treatment in a non-NHS setting but the treatment and resources will be funded by the NHS. This is a common approach where there are central policy targets in reducing waiting times, particularly for surgery.

The private sector is the industry that may provide non-clinical services such as cleaning, catering, portering or security services. The NHS or independent sector health provider may have a contract with one or more companies to provide these services.

The private sector may also be engaged in capital projects building the premises in which NHS services are provided. The private sector company may rent the premises to the NHS on a fixed-term rental agreement. This is a method by which the state can spread what would be up-front capital building costs over several decades.

The funding of continuing care is not straightforward. Where the care is provided for the prime purpose of promoting the individual's health, the care should be funded by the NHS. Where the care is provided to promote the individual's social care, that is funded by the individual. Where the individual cannot afford to pay for this care directly, there are means tested mechanisms to determine what care should be funded by social services.

Summary

- Health care is funded by the NHS.
- The NHS is funded by general taxation.
- Independent health care is funded by the individual receiving the treatment.
- Social care is funded on a means tested basis.
- Continuing care is funded by the NHS where the prime reason for needing the service is a health reason.
- The private sector may provide non-clinical services.
- The private sector may fund capital projects such as building premises leased back by the NHS.

Case study 6.2: Disputes over funding

The most important case in relation to the differences in health funding and social care funding was heard in the Court of Appeal in 1999. Where the needs of a person are assessed as being health needs, then all the care provided to that person will be funded from the NHS. Where the needs of the person are not assessed as being health needs, they can be assessed as social care needs. In these cases, the state will carry out a means test to see whether the person can pay for this care from their own financial resources. These financial resources include property ownership.

Pamela Coughlan had been injured in a road traffic accident that left her unable to live an independent life. She was cared for in a long stay hospital where her care was funded by the NHS. The Health Authority wanted to close the hospital and transfer her to a care home run by the local authority. If this happened she would be means tested as her care would in future be funded by social services. She objected to this and took the case to court. She argued that nursing care was a key funding responsibility under the NHS Act 1977 and that this should be funded in all cases by the NHS, no matter what location it was being delivered in.

At the hearing it became clear that many Health Authorities had devised eligibility criteria by which to assess whether the needs of an individual could be decided as health or social needs. The Court of Appeal decided that NHS funding should be available where the health needs of the individual are the prime reason for needing accommodation. Even where a person was living in a care home, if the health needs of the person were the prime reason for being there, the whole funding should be provided by the NHS.

Continued

As a result of this case, the Government introduced legislation that makes clear that local authorities are no longer able to provide or fund nursing care (section 49, Health and Social Care Act 2001).

R v. *North and East Devon Health Authority ex parte Coughlan* (2000)

Quality standards

The setting of standards used to be carried out directly by the Department of Health. Since 1997 a new approach has been taken to create arm's length bodies who set the standards to be met and carry out inspections to measure those standards. These agencies have powers to impose restrictions on premises where standards have fallen.

This section sets out a brief review of the main agencies that exist in England.

The Healthcare Commission

The Healthcare Commission exists to promote improvement in the quality of health care in England and Wales. In England this includes the regulation of the acute independent health care sector. It has a statutory remit to carry out inspections of every NHS facility, under the Health and Social Care (Community Health and Standards) Act 2003.

The NHS has published standards that have to be met by each NHS body, as well as developmental standards that have to be met by each body. A report is published by the Healthcare Commission giving a rating of the performance of that NHS facility. This enables the population to see how well their local NHS is performing against a national average. Financial incentives are linked to this rating.

In Wales, the Healthcare Inspectorate Wales is responsible for the local inspection and investigation of Welsh NHS bodies. The private health care sector in Wales is regulated by the Care Standards Inspectorate for Wales.

The Commission for Social Care Inspection

The Commission for Social Care Inspection (CSCI) is the body that regulates social care and the independent sector in continuing care. It provides this regulation by a system of licensing. Each provider that wants to provide this service will have to apply for a licence and be subject to annual inspection for renewal of the licence. CSCI can bring emergency powers into play where it believes that the standard of care being provided may harm the residents. Further standards set by CSCI regulate the quality of managers and the standards of qualification in management. In this manner, CSCI acts as a regulator of both settings and people.

CSCI carries out the following activities:

- Local inspections to compare all social care organizations – public, private, and voluntary – against national standards and publish reports.
- Registering services that meet national minimum standards.
- Inspections of local social service authorities.
- Publishing an annual report to Parliament on national progress on social care and an analysis of where resources have been spent.
- Validating all published performance assessment statistics on social care.
- Publishing the star ratings for social services authorities.

The National Institute for Clinical Excellence

The National Institute for Clinical Excellence (NICE) is part of the NHS. It is the independent organisation responsible for providing national guidance on treatments and care for people using the NHS in England and Wales. Where this guidance exists, it is likely to outweigh any existing guidance issued by a single regulator for a professional group.

NICE guidance is developed using the expertise of the NHS and wider health care community including NHS staff, health care professionals, patients and carers, industry and the academic community. This guidance is intended for health care professionals, patients and their carers to help them make decisions about treatment and health care.

Currently, NICE produces three kinds of guidance:

- Technology appraisals – guidance on the use of new and existing medicines and treatments within the NHS in England and Wales.
- Clinical guidelines – guidance on the appropriate treatment and care of people with specific diseases and conditions within the NHS in England and Wales.
- Interventional procedures – guidance on whether interventional procedures used for diagnosis or treatment are safe enough and work well enough for routine use in England, Wales and Scotland.

The National Patient Safety Agency

The National Patient Safety Agency (NPSA) is a Special Health Authority created to co-ordinate the efforts of all those involved in health care, and more importantly to learn from patient safety incidents occurring in the NHS. The NPSA will play a key role in bringing patient safety to a national level, enabling the entire NHS to learn from incidents and make itself safer and more stress-free for patients.

The NPSA has a remit to develop systems that create an early warning system for the NHS. The NPSA is required to implement changes in practices that will protect patients and support staff by minimising the possibilities for human error. For instance, clearer labelling of drugs can help reduce dispensing errors and overdosage, and tightening the procedures can minimise risk of mistakes surrounding spinal injections. The NPSA runs a mandatory reporting system for logging all failures, mistakes, errors and near misses across the health service. The approach taken by the Chief Medical Officer is to introduce a system that is blame-free and an open NHS where lessons are shared and learnt. While many nurses may feel that there are near misses in their practice that do not harm patients, the role of the agency is to assess from the data the circumstances that may contribute to practice being this close to danger.

As well as making sure that incidents are reported in the first place, the NPSA is aiming to promote an open and fair culture in hospitals and across the health service, encouraging doctors and other staff to report incidents and 'near misses' when things almost go wrong. A key aim is to encourage staff to report incidents without fear of personal reprimand and know that by sharing their experiences others will be able to learn lessons and improve patient safety. The NPSA collects reports from across the country and initiates preventative measures, so that the whole country can learn from each case and patient safety throughout the NHS will be improved every time.

Health Protection Agency

The Health Protection Agency's role involves:

- Advising government on public health protection policies and programmes.
- Delivering services and supporting the NHS and other agencies to protect people from infectious diseases, poisons, chemical and radiological hazards.
- Providing an impartial and authoritative source of information and advice to professionals and the public.
- Responding to new threats to public health.
- Providing a rapid response to health protection emergencies, including the deliberate release of biological, chemical, poisonous or radioactive substances.
- Improving knowledge of health protection through research, development and education and training.

The Health Protection Agency brings together the skills and expertise in a number of organisations to work in a more co-ordinated way, to reduce the burden and consequences of health protection threats or disease. The intention is to provide a more comprehensive and effective response to threats to the public's health.

National Service Frameworks

National Service Frameworks are developed with the assistance of an external reference group (ERG) which brings together health professionals, service users and carers, health service managers, partner agencies and other advocates. ERGs adopt an inclusive process to engage the full range of views. The Department of Health supports the ERGs and manages the overall process.

The role of National Service Frameworks is to:

• set national standards and identify key interventions for a defined service or care group
• put in place strategies to support implementation
• establish ways to ensure progress within an agreed time scale
• form one of a range of measures to raise quality and decrease variations in service.

There will usually be only one new framework a year. The rolling programme of National Service Frameworks was started in 1998 and now covers:

• coronary heart disease
• cancer
• paediatric intensive care
• mental health
• older people
• diabetes
• long-term conditions
• renal services
• children
• involvement of the pharmaceutical industry.

Clinical governance

Clinical governance is the system through which NHS organisations are accountable for continuously improving the quality of their services and safeguarding high standards of care, by creating an environment in which clinical excellence will flourish. Clinical governance is about changing the way people work, demonstrating that effective teamwork is as important to high quality care as risk management and clinical effectiveness.

The NHS Clinical Governance Support Team (CGST) runs a series of programmes to support the implementation of clinical governance.

These programmes enable a wide variety of NHS organisations to involve staff and patients in improving services. Development programmes involve implementing clinical governance at a number of levels.

Summary

- Standard setting by agencies is a new approach to the NHS and independent sector.
- Quality is a key feature of the health system and a main principle of the arm's length bodies.
- Many new bodies have been created over the past seven years with different functions in relation to quality.
- These bodies have powers to set standards, inspect premises and impose sanctions.
- Each agency has a different function that sets standards from a different perspective.
- The principle of arm's length agencies to set standards of quality is likely to remain a feature of the UK health system.

Application to accountability

The health service is a complex structure. It consists of different types of services that are provided in different ways and may be financed in different ways. This chapter has set out the main components of the health service in the UK. The reality of devolution means that while the services will be the same in each country, the structures that provide those services may have different names and slightly different functions.

In an assessment of accountability in nursing practice, it is necessary to understand which structure exists in providing any particular service in order to find out whether there are particular limits or boundaries on the extent of service that is provided.

The rights to treatment and care are set out in legislation. The sources of funding for treatment and care are also set out in legislation, and the interpretations of these rights have been considered by the courts.

In an assessment of accountability in nursing practice, particularly where funding and resources are identified as a limitation, it is important to assess whether the courts have already considered this particular issue in the past.

Agencies have different functions in raising quality across the health care system, depending on the reason for their existence. Each of the agencies described above has a different function, but they may all ask about similar situations at the same time in order to carry out their role. This is because the state has determined that different measures of quality in health care are needed and are to be carried out by different regulatory bodies.

In an assessment of accountability, there may be situations where a nurse is inspected by different bodies for different reasons. For example, a nurse working in the NHS in England will be aware that the Healthcare Commission is about to visit. At the same time, the National Patient Safety Agency may be making a visit to discuss ways of ensuring that electrical wiring is safe in theatre settings so that the risk of any harm to staff or patients is removed.

By now, you should be able to:

- describe the different components of a health service
- link the components in relation to your nursing practice
- assess the rights to treatment and resources
- describe the different agencies in England that set quality standards
- be confident about the role of nursing in the health service.

Summary

- There are different structures for health care in each UK country as a result of devolution.
- Funding and access to resources will be decided in legislation and clarified by court decisions.
- Regulatory bodies set standards for the systems of healthcare.

Useful websites

Scottish Executive Health Department: www.show.scot.nhs.uk/sehd
Department of Health in England: www.dh.gov.uk
National Assembly of Wales health department: www.wales.gov.uk/subihealth/nad
Northern Ireland Department of Health, Social Services and Public Safety: www.dhsspsni.gov.uk
NHS Direct: www.nhsdirect.nhs.uk
NHS Direct in Wales: www.nhsdirect.wales.nhs.uk
Healthcare Commission: www.healthcarecommission.org.uk
Commission for Social Care Inspection: www.csci.org.uk
National Institute for Clinical Excellence: www.nice.org.uk
Health Protection Agency: www.phls.co.uk
Clinical Governance Support Group: www.cgsupport.org
National Patient Safety Agency: www.npsa.nhs.uk
National Service Frameworks: www.dh.gov.uk

References

Health and Social Care Act 2001. The Stationery Office, London.
Health and Social Care (Community Health and Standards) Act 2003. The Stationery Office, London.
NHS Act 1977. The Stationery Office, London.

Department of Health (2000) *NHS Plan: A Plan for Investment, A Plan for Reform.* The Stationery Office, London.

Road Traffic (NHS Charges) Act 1999. The Stationery Office, London.

R v. *Cambridge Health Authority ex parte B* [1995] 2 All ER 129.

R v. *North and East Devon Health Authority ex parte Coughlan* [2000] 3 All ER 850.

Structures: Rights and Redress

Learning objectives

This chapter considers the place of human rights in nursing, and assesses some of the more pertinent articles from the European Convention of Human Rights. It also considers the rights of patients in the UK making a complaint, and the systems that exist to examine systematic errors in the health service.

The learning objectives for this chapter are to:

- place human rights in the context of nursing practice
- describe the European institutions that deal with human rights
- consider the main articles of the European Convention of Human Rights in the context of health care
- assess the role of inquiries into health care investigation
- understand the different stages for considering complaints about health care
- describe the role of the Ombudsman in patient complaints
- assess the role of the coroner
- review the rights of nurses in whistleblowing
- understand the process for handling a public inquiry.

Introduction

Human rights are now incorporated directly into nursing practice because the European rights that have existed over 50 years have been absorbed into UK legislation. The extent to which patients and nurses can rely on their legal human rights in relation to health care is being explored through the courts.

As the relationship between nurses and patients shifts to ensure the patient becomes the centre of the health service, there has been a greater interest in the ways that patients can ask questions about their health care. This has led to a review of the NHS complaints structure. The Ombudsman can hear complaints about health care once they have been through the NHS complaints systems. Where a patient dies, the role of the coroner in investigating the cause of death becomes important.

Wider systematic problems that take place in the health service can be identified by the nurse and there are mechanisms that allow the nurse to raise concerns where these are not being addressed in the workplace. In extreme cases, a public inquiry can be set up by Government to investigate wider issues that may require wholesale reform.

Human rights

The intensity and scope of the state-sponsored violence of the Holocaust in the middle of the twentieth century led directly to the agreement in Europe that a system was needed by which the sovereign right of any state could be open to scrutiny by other states. The aim was to create an international framework, resulting in the European Convention of Human Rights, with the UK being its first signatory in 1950 (European Convention, 1950).

The European Convention of Human Rights is a series of Articles and Protocols, each giving a set of obligations to the countries that have signed up to the Convention. Where any citizen in one of these countries believes that the rights have not been upheld by the state, that citizen can ask an independent court outside his or her country to investigate. Where the court agrees with the citizen, the country will have to change the system so that it behaves in a way that is consistent with the Convention.

Social and economic rights are not covered in the Convention, because these rights were not the most urgent at the time the Convention was created. As a result there is no Article that gives a right to the provision of basic health care. Even though the UK was one of the first signatories to this Convention, it only incorporated the rights into domestic law in the Human Rights Act 1998. This Act means that any legislation in the UK must now be considered in the light of the Convention. It also provides the citizens of the UK with a right to argue in court that any of the rights in the Convention have been broken.

Nursing has a fundamental commitment to the wellbeing of the patient and to a professional practice based on codes of ethics. The International Council of Nurses (ICN) has a Position Statement on Nurses and Human Rights (1998) which sets out a nurse's responsibilities towards human rights. The ICN points out that nurses have an individual responsibility but they can be more effective if they approach human rights issues as a group.

Human rights institutions in Europe

The European Convention of Human Rights
The Convention, which came into effect on 4 October 1950, is an agreement by which member States of the Council of Europe agree to protect fundamental human rights.

The European Commission of Human Rights
The European Commission of Human Rights is an independent international body set up under the European Convention of Human Rights. Each member state of the Council of Europe that signs the Convention can place one member on the Commission. The members of the Commission are independent of governments and do not have any duty to represent their country on the Commission. In this way, the Commission can be representative of all the countries that have signed the Convention.

The role of the European Commission of Human Rights is to process and mediate in the complaints made by an individual that his or her member state has violated rights or freedoms recognised under the Convention. Complaints can come from an individual, groups of people or non-governmental organisations. The person making the complaint must claim that a public body of a member state has broken one of the freedoms or rights in the Convention, and that the person complaining has suffered as a result. The Commission can only deal with complaints about matters that are the responsibility of a public authority. The Commission cannot deal with complaints against private persons or organisations. This means that complaints can be made about the NHS but cannot be made about private health care providers.

The European Court of Human Rights
The European Court of Human Rights in Strasbourg will hear the cases that cannot be mediated. These cases are heard in public. The Court of Human Rights will give a judgement on whether or not a violation of the Convention has taken place. The court's decision is final and is binding on the country concerned. The court can order that a payment of compensation is made to the individual. Where there has been a breach in human rights, the country will generally have to consider whether to alter its own law or administrative procedures as a result of the court's decision. Other countries may want to consider whether the judgement has an effect on their own law.

Main articles of the European Convention for the Protection of Human Rights and Fundamental Freedoms

Article 2: Right to life

Article 2 provides that 'everyone's right to life shall be protected by law. No one shall be deprived of his life intentionally save in the execution of a sentence of a court following his conviction of a crime for which this penalty is provided by law.' It is important to note that this does not say 'everyone has a right to life'. This Article provides that the law will be used to protect life. Euthanasia and abortion are therefore not automatically prohibited by this Article.

In *Widmer* v. *Switzerland* (1993), the Commission found that allowing a person to die by withholding treatment may be permitted. However this distinction in law is based on the notion of passive acts (not giving the treatment) and does not allow active acts (deliberately giving someone an overdose). It is an accepted part of civil law that an adult of sound mind has full autonomy to decide not to have further treatment even where the outcome is that he will die. His reasons for refusal do not have to be rational.

In *LCB* v. *United Kingdom* (1998) the case concerned a child who was at risk of developing leukaemia from her father who had been exposed to radiation while working on Christmas Island. The court accepted the principle that if the state knew or ought to have known of a particular life-threatening risk, it should warn those affected. This suggests that the Article places a burden on health bodies to make the public aware of environmental risks.

Article 3: Prohibition of Torture

Article 3 provides that 'No one shall be subjected to torture or to inhuman or degrading treatment or punishment'. In a very early decision the court considered the definition of 'degrading', and found that treatment can only be degrading if it grossly humiliates the victim or drives him to act against his will or conscience.

In *Tanko* v. *Finland* (1994) the court decided that a failure to provide proper medical treatment could be a breach of Article 3. It is not clear what would be covered by the phrase 'proper medical treatment'. It may cover matters such as inadequate pain relief or being made to wait on a trolley in an accident and emergency department.

The court has used Article 3 to find a breach of the Convention for a failure to provide treatment under the NHS. In the case of *D* v. *United Kingdom* (1994) the court found that to send the man who had AIDS to St Kitts where there was no provision for his treatment amounted to 'acute mental and physical suffering'.

The rights of children will be important under this Article. In one significant case, *A* v. *United Kingdom* (1998), the court found that the parental right to smack a child was not an appropriate exemption to this Article. The court found that parental smacking was incompatible with the positive duty to prevent degrading treatment.

Treatment of babies and young children with drugs which have not been tested may also amount to a breach under Article 3.

Article 4: Prohibition of Slavery And Forced Labour
The main aspect of Article 4 is that 'No one shall be required to perform forced or compulsory labour'.

In the case of *Iverson* v. *Norway* (1963) a dentist challenged a law in Norway that required him to work for two years in the public dental service. The Commission found that the application was not admissible and the case did not go to the court. The Commission found that the service 'was for a short period, provided favourable remuneration, did not involve any diversion from chosen professional work . . . and did not involve any discriminatory, arbitrary or punitive application'.

Article 6: Right to A Fair Trial
Article 6 provides that everyone is entitled to a fair and public hearing within a reasonable time by an independent and impartial tribunal established by law. There must be a guarantee of a fair trial in any civil or criminal proceedings. This means that the NMC and other regulatory bodies will need to make sure that their procedures are compatible with the Article, otherwise anyone affected would have the ability to challenge the procedure.

The NHS complaints procedures will be subject to the requirements of Article 6 and the NHS will have to ensure that the processes used at all levels of complaints handling are independent and impartial, particularly where a complaint about the provision of treatment is made. It will also be important that people being refused NHS treatment are given reasons for this which are compatible with Article 6.

In a case concerning a GP (*Trivedi* v. *United Kingdom* (1997)) the GP was convicted of theft for claiming payments for visits to a patient which were not made. The patient made statements about the extent of the visits but his illness meant that he was unable to give evidence at the trial. The judge took the statements and used these in the trial, leading to the GP's conviction. The GP took his case to the European Court of Human Rights claiming that there had been a breach of Article 6(3) in that he had been unable to challenge the patient. His case failed. The court found that the judge had made extensive investigations into the patient's condition and that the judge was also able to rely on prescription sheets written by the GP which supported the patient's statement.

Article 8: Right to Respect for Private and Family Life
Article 8 guarantees the right to respect for private and family life, home and correspondence. It has been interpreted in a variety of ways

and for a variety of situations. There are some limits on the extent to which this right has to be promoted, including where there is a need to protect health or morals. The right is watered down by Article 8(2) which allows interference with the right where it is 'necessary in a democratic society' in a number of situations.

Article 8 protects privacy, family life and home life. The right to privacy has several aspects touching on physical privacy, for example mixed sex wards and the use of surveillance equipment; and on personal privacy for example the provision of personal information and issues of sexual orientation.

The Court of Appeal directly applied the rights in Article 8 in the case of R v. *North and East Devon Health Authority ex parte Coughlan* (1999). Pamela Coughlan was a resident in an NHS hospital. The Health Authority wanted to close the hospital and move her to a nursing home. They had made an oral promise to her when she moved into the hospital several years earlier that this would be her 'home for life'. The Court of Appeal held that the promise should be protected and that a decision to move her to a different home breached her rights under Article 8. It did not matter whether it was reasonable for the Health Authority to consider closure of the hospital, for the breach of her rights to occur.

In the case of *Guerra* v. *Italy* (1998) the court found that there had been an infringement of Article 8 and Article 2 where the authorities failed to take practical measures to lower the risk posed by a chemical factory to those who were living one kilometre away. There was a failure to provide essential information about the environment.

Article 8(2) does allow some justification for compulsory treatment. In *Acmanne* v. *Belgium* (1983) the court found that compulsory tuberculosis screening was an interference of private life but was justified as necessary to protect health.

Article 12: Right to Marry

Men and women of marriageable age have the right to marry and to found a family, according to the national laws governing the exercise of this right. The rights and freedoms are subject to domestic law existing in the individual member states. This means, for example, that the different age limits at which men and women can marry do not need to be similar across all countries which have signed up to the Convention.

Where there are already national laws in place regarding marriage the court will not seek to overturn those. In the case of *Johnston* v. *Ireland* (1987), the court found that the laws in Ireland which prevent divorce, and which also prohibit divorced people from remarrying, are lawful. Where countries prohibit marriage by homosexuals or transsexuals, the court will not overturn this either.

Convention rights incorporated into the Human Rights Act 1998

Table 7.1 lists Articles in the Convention and the rights they protect which have been incorporated into the Human Rights Act 1998.

Table 7.1 List of Convention Articles in the Human Rights Act 1998.

Article in the Convention	Human right protected
2	Right to life
3	Right not to be subjected to torture or inhuman treatment
4	Right to freedom from slavery or forced labour
5	Right to liberty and security of person
6	Right to a fair trial
7	Right to no punishment without law
8	Right to respect for private and family life, home and correspondence
9	Right to freedom of thought, conscience and religion
10	Right to freedom of expression
11	Right to freedom of peaceful assembly and freedom of association
12	Right to marry and found a family
14	Right not to be discriminated against in the enjoyment of the rights and freedoms in the Act
16	Exception to rights in Articles 10, 11 and 14 in relation to restricting the political activities of aliens
17	Prohibition of abuse of Convention rights
18	Limitation on use of restrictions on rights permitted by the Convention
The First Protocol Article 1	Right to peaceful enjoyment of possessions
The First Protocol, Article 2	Right to education
The First Protocol, Article 3	Right to free elections
The Sixth Protocol, Articles 1 and 2	Abolition of the death penalty except in times of war or imminent threat of war

Redress in health care

Complaints

Patient complaints have become a recognised part of nursing practice in health care. There are now systems in place which allow patients to make complaints about their care in the NHS and the independent sector. There is nothing to stop the individual patient making a complaint about fitness to practice to any of the professional regulatory bodies where the care from the clinical professional has fallen below the standards acceptable to that body.

Where the patient has been injured as a result of treatment, it is possible for him to make a claim to the NHS Litigation Authority for a claim in negligence. The NHS Litigation Authority handles clinical negligence claims and publishes information on risk management.

In each NHS Trust in England there are Patient Liaison and Advocacy Services that assist patients who want to make a complaint. The Citizens Advice Bureau will also assist anyone with the process of the healthcare complaints system.

The process for dealing with complaints in the NHS and the independent sector in England is as follows.

First stage: local resolution

Anyone who wants to make a complaint about any aspect of NHS or independent sector treatment that has been received or any treatment that has been refused can make a complaint. This also applies to family members and advocates on behalf of that individual. The first stage is for that person to go directly to the GP, hospital, clinic or Trust concerned, and ask for a copy of their complaints procedure. This system covers any care given in the NHS, even where it is provided in an independent sector setting.

Most health settings will have a designated member of staff who is the complaints manager, with the intention that the majority of complaints will be resolved at this stage.

Second stage: independent review

Where the complaint cannot be resolved at local level, the next stage is to pass the NHS or independent sector complaint to the Healthcare Commission for an independent review.

The Healthcare Commission will take over the handling of any complaint and act as a second tier in the process (Healthcare Commission, 2004). When a complaint is received by the Healthcare Commission, it will:

- Appoint a case manager who will check that all relevant information is available.
- Carry out an initial review to decide whether it is both possible and appropriate for the Healthcare Commission to investigate the case. If the NHS procedure is not yet finished, for example, the Healthcare Commission will request that this is completed before taking further action. The documents needed for this review will include the medical and nursing records and the appropriate consent forms. The case manager may call for independent expert evidence. Generally the initial review will be completed within 10 days of all the relevant information being available.
- Carry out an investigation under terms of reference which are agreed between the individual complaining and the health care provider. An independent expert advisor will assist the investigation. The case manager may interview witnesses. A report will be written to be agreed with the parties and this will contain recommendations about action to be taken. The investigation usually takes six months.

- Hold a panel if the individual making the complaint is unhappy with the outcome. The panel will have a chair and two panel members and will produce a report of the decisions and recommendations made. The panel will normally complete its task within four months.

The individual making the complaint can make a further complaint to the Health Service Ombudsman if he or she is unhappy about the decisions made by the Healthcare Commission.

Third stage: Health Service Ombudsman
Where the patient feels that the complaint should be taken further, she or he can ask the Health Service Ombudsman to investigate. The Health Service Ombudsman can investigate complaints about clinical procedures. The Ombudsman's function is to check that the Government has acted fairly in its administration.

Summary

- Complaints are now an accepted part of the health service in the NHS and the independent sector.
- Complaints about clinical negligence can be made to the NHS Litigation Authority.
- Patient advisors and organisations like the Citizens Advice Bureau assist patients in the complaints process.
- There is a staged process for making complaints in health care.

The Ombudsman

The Health Service Ombudsman for England investigates complaints against NHS Health Authorities and Trusts, Primary Care Trusts and primary care practitioners in England, and also investigates complaints about independent providers of health care funded by the NHS.

The Ombudsman accepts cases directly from complainants and has jurisdiction over the NHS with regard to:

- maladministration
- failure to provide a service
- failures in providing a service, including the exercise of clinical judgement
- the Code of Practice on Openness in the NHS (Department of Health, 1995).

A set of papers can be sent to the Ombudsman only after the NHS complaints procedure has been completed. This means that a referral will take place after the complaint has been investigated by the Healthcare Commission.

Where NHS providers refuse to take part in an aspect of the complaints procedure, that will be enough for the patient or his family to go to the Ombudsman. When the Ombudsman has completed her investigations, she may make a report to the House of Commons Select Committee. This causes considerable publicity and means that the NHS provider is almost certain to take immediate steps to change their procedures.

Summary

- The Ombudsman is appointed by the Queen and reports to Parliament.
- The Ombudsman carries out independent investigations into maladministration by Government departments and public bodies.
- The investigation is private.
- Different Ombudsmen cover England, Wales, Scotland and Northern Ireland.
- They considers hardship or injustice resulting from failure to provide a service or from failure in service.
- The Ombudsman cannot consider complaints about private health care, NHS personnel matters or matters which the complainant intends to take to court.
- The Ombudsman makes recommendations which are usually accepted by the Government.

Activity

Look at the website for the Ombudsman at www.ombudsman.org.uk and look at the most recent annual report on health care. What was the most striking feature of this report for you?

Coroner

The Home Office has responsibility for coroners. Their fees and salaries are paid by local authorities. The Coroner's Act 1988 is the legislation that sets out the functions and duties of a coroner. Barristers, solicitors or doctors can apply to become coroners when they have been in practice for over five years. Some become full-time coroners, while others work on a part-time basis.

The coroner responds to all deaths that are reported to the coroner's office. At present this accounts for just over one-third of all deaths. In the light of the case of Harold Shipman and the outcome of the public inquiry, there may be an overhaul of the system by which deaths are reported to the coroner. This would allow an assessment of patterns of death in hospital and the community.

Coroners investigate deaths which are violent, unnatural or of a sudden or unexpected nature. Deaths that take place during an operation or due to an industrial disease will also be referred to the coroner. The coroner will establish the medical cause of death, generally by a post-mortem. This will be done by a pathologist of the coroner's choosing. If the post-mortem is inconclusive, an inquest will be held.

An inquest is a public hearing which takes evidence from witnesses and experts to get information that will help the coroner decide the medical cause of death. It is an inquiry into who has died, and how, when and where the death occurred. An inquest will be held with a jury where the death occurred in prison, in custody, at work or if further deaths could occur in similar circumstances.

The verdicts that can be given at an inquest include:

- natural causes
- accident
- suicide
- unlawful killing
- lawful killing
- industrial disease
- open verdict.

Summary

- The coroner investigates unexplained deaths.
- The functions of the coroner are set out in legislation.
- Where a death is referred to the coroner, a post-mortem will take place.
- An inquest may be needed to find out the cause of death.
- Some inquests are heard with a jury.
- There is a range of verdicts that can be made at an inquest.

Whistleblowing

The Public Interest Disclosure Act 1998 protects nurses who speak out against wrongdoing and abuse. It applies to nurses working in both the NHS and the independent sector, to agency nurses and to nurse students in the workplace. Confidentiality clauses in contracts and severance agreements, which conflict with the provisions of the Act, are now unlawful.

Government guidance

The Department of Health has issued guidance which applies to England (Department of Health, 1999). Called *Whistleblowing in the NHS*, it requires that all NHS Trusts should ensure that they have policies in place for whistleblowing. A senior manager or non-executive director should be designated with specific responsibility for addressing concerns raised in the organisation. The guidance recognises that there are 'powerful disincentives' in place that could prevent staff from raising concerns about problems in the workplace. The guidance also recognises that the failure to speak up early enough has led to incidents which could have been prevented, so encourages the reporting of concerns to ensure high public confidence in the NHS.

NMC Code of Professional Conduct

The NMC expects nurses to report concerns about levels of care that appear to be creating difficulties. Clause 8.3 states that 'Where you cannot remedy circumstances in the environment of care that could jeopardise standards of practice, you must report them to a senior person with sufficient authority to manage them and also, in the case of midwifery, to the supervisor of midwives. This must be supported by a written record.' Clause 8.4 states that 'When working as a manager, you have a duty toward patients and clients, colleagues, the wider community and the organisation in which you and your colleagues work. When facing professional dilemmas, your first consideration in all activities must be the interests and safety of patients.'

Employment

Where a nurse considers that there are issues of concern in the workplace the following processes should be followed:

- Consult local whistleblowing procedures from the employer.
- Where possible, raise the issue internally first with a line manager or a senior colleague or clinical supervisor.
- Talking through the issues is a good way to clarify what action needs to be taken.
- Keep a diary of significant incidents and all conversations, and notes of actions, in relation to each incident.
- Where the nurse believes that no action has been taken to resolve the issue, he or she should put their concerns in writing to the Chief Executive.
- It is advisable to consult with the relevant professional organisation.
- Where there is no satisfactory answer from the Chief Executive, the nurse should take advice about the appropriate external bodies to which to report the concerns, in order to satisfy the steps in the legislation.

Summary

- There are legal rights for a nurse to raise concerns about the standard of health care
- These rights are reinforced by the NMC Code of Professional Conduct.
- Nurses who want to raise concerns should be clear about the process to be used.

Public inquiries

The Government will set up a public inquiry when there has been an incident (generally involving death) which raises questions about wider health or safety issues. There is a defined process that will take place for any public inquiry, as set out below. The public inquiry is funded by the Government and is headed by an independent chair of impartial reputable standing, usually a judge. The recommendations made by the inquiry have to be considered by the Government, who will usually make changes to the structure of the wider system as a result.

Major public inquiries over the past decade include:

- The Bristol Royal Infirmary Inquiry
- The Victoria Climbie Inquiry
- The Harold Shipman Inquiry.

Announcement of an inquiry

Public inquiries are usually triggered by a death or broad trauma in circumstances where public bodies have been involved. The announcement of a public inquiry will be made by the relevant Secretary of State who will publish the terms of reference and the names of the chair and team who will be asked to carry out the investigation. The final report and recommendations are given to the Secretary of State who publishes this along with the Government's response to the recommendations.

Phase One

The inquiry team will appoint lawyers who will contact persons who can provide evidence (written or oral) about the facts of the death or trauma. These people will have been directly involved in the incident. They may require legal representation.

Phase Two

The inquiry team will place the facts in the broader context of society at the time, and to do this they take evidence from professional groups on current policy at that time. The inquiry team look for gaps in the public service and assess what measures could be taken to prevent a similar incident.

Publication

The inquiry team present the report to the Secretary of State. This sets out the detail of what happened (phase one evidence), the context in which it happened (phase two investigation), and makes recommendations as to how the Government can make changes so that the system can be improved.

Government's response

The Secretary of State publishes the report in the House of Commons. The Secretary of State is required to give the Government's response to the recommendations. The Secretary of State may ask for views and comments on the recommendations before making the Government's response.

Application to accountability

There are many different sources of rights and redress in health care. This chapter has set out the most important for both patients and nurses. This will enable nurses to engage more proactively in systems for assessing the issues raised by patients about the standard of health care received.

The structures for ensuring that patients have access to information about their health care continue to develop, so it is important that nurses are confident about current systems in order to be able to influence future developments. This will be to the benefit of both patients and nurses.

By now, you should be able to:

- be confident about different types of rights and redress in the health service
- set out the key components of the European Convention of Human Rights
- apply rights and redress in the context of nursing practice
- understand that rights and redress are part of the wider accountability in nursing.

Useful websites

European Court of Human Rights: www.echr.coe.int
International Council of Nurses: www.icn.ch
Healthcare Commission: www.healthcarecommission.org.uk
Citizens Advice Bureau: www.adviceguide.org.uk
NHS Litigation Authority: www.nhsla.com
Health Service Ombudsman: www.ombudsman.org.uk
Home Office: www.homeoffice.gov.uk
Reports from the Public Inquiry on Harold Shipman: www.the-shipman-inquiry.org.uk

References

A v. *United Kingdom* [1998] ECHR 85.
Acmanne v. *Belgium* (1983) 40 DR 251.

Coroner's Act 1988. The Stationery Office, London.

D v. *United Kingdom* (1994) 24 EHRR 423.

Department of Health (1995) *The Code of Practice on Openness in the NHS*. NHS Executive.

Department of Health (1999) *Whistleblowing in the NHS* (HSG 1999/198). NHS Executive. The Stationery Office, London.

Department of Health (2001) *Report of the Public Inquiry into Children's Heart Surgery at Bristol Royal Infirmary 1984-1995: Learning from Bristol*. The Stationery Office, London.

European Convention for the Protection of Human Rights and Fundamental Freedoms (1950). Council of Europe, Strasbourg.

Guerra v. *Italy* (1998) 26 EHRR 357.

Healthcare Commission (2004), *Unhappy with the way your complaint has been handled by the NHS? Contact the Healthcare Commission*. Healthcare Commission, London.

Human Rights Act 1998. The Stationery Office, London.

International Council of Nurses (1998) *Position Statement on Nurses and Human Rights*. ICN, Geneva.

Iverson v. *Norway* (1963) 6 Yearbook 278.

Johnston v. *Ireland* (1987) 9 EHRR 203.

LCB v. *United Kingdom* [1998] TLR 381.

Nursing and Midwifery Council (2002) *Code of Professional Conduct*. NMC, London.

Public Interest Disclosure Act 1998. The Stationery Office, London.

R v. *North and East Devon Health Authority ex parte Coughlan* [2000] 3 All ER 850.

Tanko v. *Finland* (1994) Application No. 23634/94 (unreported) E Comm HR.

Third Report of the Shipman Enquiry (2003) Command Paper CM5854. The Stationery Office, London.

Trivedi v. *United Kingdom* (1997) EHRLR 521.

Victoria Climbie Inquiry Report (2003) The Stationery Office, London.

Widmer v. *Switzerland* (1993) Application No. 20527/92 (unreported) E Comm HR.

Concepts: Negligence

Learning objectives

Negligence is an area of nursing practice that can strike horror into the heart of the most robust nurse. The idea that you may have to appear in court to justify your action in front of a patient who has been determined enough to pursue a case can be a mechanism for creating the most defensive approach to nursing practice.

In reality few of the cases that are started reach court. One of the objectives of this chapter is to set out the framework that exists in negligence, so you can see that reaching court can be a major achievement in itself for a patient. Most patients take a case in negligence because they have been frustrated in getting an explanation for what went wrong, or they want to make sure the same issue does not happen to anyone else.

The learning objectives for this chapter are to:

- have a clear understanding about the principles that underpin negligence
- be confident about time limits and defences to negligence
- place negligence in the context of the NMC Code of Professional Conduct
- understand the different standards of care required by the law and by the NMC
- be able to understand the features of compensation
- be confident about nursing practice in the context of a potential negligence claim
- place negligence in the framework of accountability.

Introduction

Negligence is a civil tort. If nurses give care that does not meet appropriate standards, they may be held liable for negligence. Negligence is a basic part of the legal framework that applies to nursing practice. There is no Act of Parliament that sets out the principles for negligence. However, the case law that has been developed in the courts has created a principled approach in law.

In an action for negligence, the following principles must be established:

- The nurse (defendant) owed a duty of care to the patient (claimant).
- The nurse broke that duty by failing to act as a reasonable nurse.
- The patient/client was injured as a result of the nurse breaking that duty.
- There is compensation that can be paid as a result of the negligence.

Each one of these aspects must be proved before a claim of negligence can be successful. If at any stage one of the issues is not proved, the whole case of negligence will fail.

There have been complaints that the current system of negligence is not helpful to patients who have been injured. The complaints are generally focused on three types of issue:

- the amount of time taken to finish a negligence action
- the cost of taking a case to court and the risk of having to pay the legal costs of the other side
- the only remedy is cash, which does not guarantee the same problem will not affect another patient.

Nurses are responsible for performing all procedures correctly and exercising professional judgement as they carry out their own tasks and those ordered by a doctor. Any nurse who does not meet accepted standards of practice or who performs duties in a careless fashion, runs the risk of being negligent.

It is also important to consider that in health care, genuine accidents happen that are not negligent. Where the health outcome is different from what had been expected, this does not mean that a negligence action will be successful. The law will not deal with genuine accidents in the context of a negligence claim. The key issue in a case of negligence is that another person can be shown to be at fault for the outcome. Where there is no one to blame for the outcome, there can be no negligence.

Summary

- There is no Act of Parliament that defines negligence.
- A set of principles have been decided by case law that must succeed for a claim in negligence to succeed.

- Each principle has to be proved before a claim in negligence will succeed.
- Negligence has been criticised for the time, cost and remedies that are involved.
- Genuine accidents should not be confused with negligence.
- The key issue in negligence is that a person or a system is at fault.

The first principle: duty of care

This first principle of negligence is that a duty of care must be owed by one person to another. This is based on the ideal that a duty to take care is owed by one person to another where there is a connection that can be described as a neighbour principle. If this duty does not exist, there cannot be a claim in negligence. This principle was based on the case of *Donoghue* v. *Stephenson* in 1932, set out in more detail in Case Study 8.1.

In health care the duty of care is usually straightforward and not an issue of contention. A person receiving treatment from a doctor or nurse will be owed a duty of care by that professional. If the person has treatment using equipment which is faulty, the manufacturer of that equipment will owe a duty of care to the patient.

How far the duty of care can be extended is an issue that has been tested in the courts. Where a doctor discharges a patient with an infectious illness and others are then infected, the courts have found that the doctor owed a duty of care to those who became infected, even though they were not his patients (*Evans* v. *Liverpool Corp* (1906)).

A duty of care may exist for those who witness a traumatic event in which others are injured. The courts have had to consider principles of public policy in these cases but have also had to consider how far a duty of care can be given to those who are not in the direct consideration of the person causing the injury. In most cases, the duty of care will be directly owed by a nurse to a patient, or by a bank manager to a client, or by a kettle manufacturer to the end consumers. However, in a very limited instance, the courts have found that an indirect duty of care can be owed to those who witness the injury taking place. Case Study 8.2 sets out these principles in more detail.

Where a person invites others to come to his premises, there is a responsibility on the occupier to make sure the premises are safe. This can apply to those who have health facilities in hospitals or in surgeries. It can also apply to the individual patient in the community who asks for home visits from a doctor or nurse. All occupiers have a duty of care to those who are invited to their property. This duty of care has also been included in legislation that deals with the responsibilities of those who own property, the Occupier's Liability Act 1984.

Summary

- The duty of care is based on the 'neighbour' principle.
- In healthcare the duty of care is between the patient and the health service, including the persons treating that individual.
- The duty of care can extend to the manufacturers of equipment in relation to the end consumers.
- The duty of care may be extended to people who are indirectly affected by an event, through nervous shock.
- Those who occupy property have a duty of care to their visitors in case law as well as in legislation.

Case study 8.1: The duty of care

The legal concept of a duty of care was established in the famous 1932 case of *Donoghue* v. *Stephenson*. This is often said to be the first case that law students study. The facts of the case are unusual, as the situation often is in negligence actions.

A woman and her friend went to a tea shop. The friend bought a bottle of ginger beer which the woman drank. It was produced at that time in glass opaque bottles. She could not see what was in the bottle. She became ill as a result of drinking the ginger beer. She discovered to her horror that at the bottom of the bottle were the remains of a decomposed snail. She sued the manufacturers.

The court discussed and clarified that a neighbour principle between the manufacturer and the woman meant that the manufacturer owed a duty of care to all its end consumers. The court held that the manufacturers of the ginger beer owed her a duty of care to produce an uncontaminated drink.

This principle is now the basis on which any dispute over whether a duty of care exists is decided.

Donoghue v. *Stephenson* (1932)

Case study 8.2: Extending the duty of care

The Hillsborough Disaster in 1989 was witnessed by many people on television. The FA cup semi-final was being played at the Hillsborough football ground, where many people became crushed in one end of the stadium. Family members who were watching television saw pictures of the dead and injured being carried away. They suffered psychiatric shock. They sued claiming that a duty of care was owed to them, even though they were not at the stadium.

The House of Lords held that a duty of care can exist in these circumstances but that only designated family members could claim this duty of care. It would

Continued

not be enough for a member of the general public to be able to claim a duty of care for psychiatric harm.

The House of Lords were concerned that there should be a known limit on the extent to which an indirect duty of care can be identified, so that those who are in the insurance industry can be clear about the range of risk for any activity.

Alcock v. *Chief Constable of South Yorkshire Police* (1991)

Activity

A wife received a call to say her husband was involved in an accident. She went to the Accident and Emergency Department. The clerk told her to look in cubicle 4, but did not say that her husband had died. The woman suffered psychiatric shock as a result.

Is there a duty of care in this case? If so, where does it lie? What action would you want to take to make sure it did not happen again?

The second principle: breaking the duty of care

The second principle requires that the duty of care must be broken if a negligence action is to succeed. It is broken if the standard of care is not met. The test to decide whether the duty of care is broken is based on 'the reasonable man' and what he would consider to be the reasonable standard of care in any given situation. In health cases this means that the duty of care is broken if a nurse fails to act to the standard that would have been met by a hypothetical reasonable nurse in that same situation.

This test was created in the case of *Bolam* v. *Friern Barnet Management Committee* in 1957. The rule was formulated that 'a doctor is not guilty of negligence if he has acted in accordance with a practice accepted as proper by a responsible body of medical men skilled in that particular art'. This test means that where a nurse acts in a way that would be supported by nursing opinion as being appropriate practice at that time, it is likely the court will find that she did not break her duty of care.

In practice, where this is an issue in a court case, the use of an expert witness will show the general standard of practice in nursing at the time of the incident. The fact that there is an opposing body of opinion does not automatically indicate that there has been negligence. Case study 4.3 in Chapter 4 sets out some issues to consider about being an expert witness.

Where a nurse is working at a higher level of practice, the standard to be used by the law will be that higher standard. Nurses who undertake nursing practice at a higher level will be judged by the court to be negligent if they do not achieve this and a patient is harmed. The nurse will not be able to choose to claim that she should be judged at a lower standard.

Where student nurses are providing care, they are judged by standards of an experienced nurse. This is because the courts have held that patients are entitled to care that is competent. This will mean that it is important for students to call for supervision wherever they are unclear about a procedure. Once a student is registered as a nurse, the lack of experience will not be allowed as a defence as the courts require that newly qualified nurses are expected to able to practice as if they were experienced. However, the courts have accepted that junior staff who clearly set out the limits on their competence will be recognised as having met their standard of care. The best way to do this is to ask a more experienced member of staff to check the work. It is important that the nurse challenges instructions that she believes are incorrect.

Summary

- The test for breaking the standard of care is known as 'the Bolam test'.
- The key to this test is whether the nurse was acting as a reasonable nurse.
- Nurses working at a higher standard will be judged as reasonable only if they have acted at that higher standard.
- The courts will not make allowances in standards of care for the learner or the newly qualified.
- Junior staff who seek clarification of a procedure follow their standard of care.

Case study 8.3: Breaking the duty of care

Patrick Bolitho, two years old, was admitted to hospital where he was observed by the senior sister to be having fits. Each time she observed this, she rang the House Officer. The Consultant Paediatric Registrar failed to attend the child on two occasions over the course of one day, despite being telephoned by the Paediatric Sister at 12.40 and 2.00 pm. On the third occasion the child had a fit and suffered brain damage. He later died.

The mother sued the hospital, particularly for the failure by the doctor to attend the child. The court found that the senior sister had acted in accordance with nursing opinion in the actions she took, and that she had not broken her duty of care. The court found that the failure by the doctor to attend the child was below the standard that would have been expected by a doctor, and that she had broken her duty of care to the child. This of itself does not mean that

Continued

negligence was successful, but it does show that the first two principles were proved against the doctor.

Bolitho v. *City and Hackney Health Authority* (1997)

Activity

Read the case of Bolitho available on the website www.parliament.uk (follow the link to judicial work, then to judgements for 1997). Look at when the events took place and compare this with the date of the judgement in the House of Lords. What do you think about the length of time between the two dates? Is it what you expected it might be?

The third principle: causation

One of the reasons many cases in negligence fail is because the claimant cannot show causation. This is the stage in a negligence action where the claimant must show that the injury was caused only by the failure in the duty of care. There must be a direct link between the failure and the injury. If there is no direct link, the negligence claim will fail.

A nurse may break a duty of care and the patient may be injured, but in order to establish negligence it is necessary to show a link between the two. This is known as the 'but for' test. It means that but for the break in the duty of care, there would have been no harm caused. This means that a nurse can break the standard of care by acting in a manner that is openly reckless and dangerous, but if there is no harm caused to the patient as a result, there will be no negligence. The law is not interested just in the behaviour of the nurse. The law is interested in the consequence of the behaviour.

In some cases it is so obvious that the injury was caused by the failure in standards that it is clear the causation exists. This is known as *res ipsa loquitor* (the facts speak for themselves). An example of this is where a patient suffers an infection caused by a swab that was inadvertently left in his abdomen following surgery. Cases in this category are rare.

It is for the patient or person making the claim of negligence to prove on the balance of probabilities that the link between the standard of care and the harm is proved. In most cases this will be by the use of medical expert witnesses.

The courts have also developed the principle of the 'eggshell skull' to provide that where one person is more susceptible to harm because he or she has a particular vulnerability, this cannot be dismissed just because another person would not have suffered the same harm.

Summary

- Causation must be shown, as the third principle of negligence.
- Causation is the link between the standard of care and harm to the patient.
- The nurse may behave recklessly but if there is no harm, there is no negligence.
- *Res ipsa loquitor* is where the link between the failure in standards and the cause of the harm is obvious.
- The proof of causation is on the balance of probabilities.
- A person with a particular vulnerability may be able to rely on the 'eggshell skull' rule to show causation.

Case study 8.4: Showing the link of causation

In *Barnet* v. *Chelsea and Kensington* (1968), three night-watchmen visited an accident and emergency unit in the early hours of the morning complaining of sickness and vomiting. It later transpired that their tea flasks had been laced with arsenic. The nurse in accident and emergency rang the doctor to ask for advice and was told by the doctor to inform the men to see their GP later that day. One man died before seeing his GP and his wife sued the hospital in negligence. The court found that the nurse had acted in accordance with her duty of care to the men by seeking advice from the doctor and that she had not breached her duty of care and could not be held negligent.

   The court found that the casualty doctor should have examined the men at the hospital, and that any reasonable doctor would have done so. By failing to act in accordance with the generally accepted standard, the doctor had broken his duty of care. However, the evidence showed the man would have died of poisoning in any event, even if the doctor had seen him. The failure to treat was not in itself a sufficient cause of injury (in this case, death) for a finding of negligence against the doctor.

Barnett v. *Chelsea and Kensington* (1968)

The fourth principle: compensation

The fourth principle of negligence requires that the injury can be measured so that a cash sum of compensation can be paid. There have been complaints that payment of cash is not sufficient to compensate for the harm that has been caused. Many people who sue in negligence want an apology, while others want an assurance that the system will be changed so that a similar situation will not happen again. The legal word for this compensation is damages.

The principle is that the amount of compensation should place the victim in as close as position as he would have been in just before the incident happened. Large sums will therefore be paid where the victim is very young and needs specialist care for the rest of his life.

Compensation is divided into two types:

- General damages for the pain and suffering caused. This will be calculated by reference to a text book setting out levels of value for different types of injury.
- Special damages for the financial losses suffered. This will be calculated by assessing what income, both past and future, has been lost as a result of the accident, including pension loss. Other cash payment will cover additional financial costs from the injury. If a person needs to adapt a car because of a serious back injury, the cost will be part of the claim under special damages. If he is no longer able to garden and now has to employ someone to do it, this cost will be added to the claim.

Where the injury is so severe that the victim of negligence dies, there are methods by which his or her dependent family can continue the claim and ask for compensation. This will be calculated based on the financial income and contribution to the household that the deceased person would have made.

Summary

- Compensation is made by a cash payment.
- There is no entitlement to an apology or a change in the system.
- Compensation can be for general and special damages.
- In fatal accidents, compensation can be paid to the family.

Case study 8.5: Public policy limits on compensation claims

Limits on the extent to which a person can claim cash compensation for their losses was discussed in 1999. In this case, Ms Briordy was left infertile by treatment and wanted to claim the cost of travelling to America for surrogacy treatment. Surrogacy is only allowed in the UK on an altruistic basis, and she wanted to enter into a commercial arrangement as she wanted greater guarantees that she could have a surrogate baby. The courts found that, on the grounds of public policy, it would be inappropriate to allow her the cost of this overseas treatment when it had been outlawed by Parliament.

Briordy v. *St Helens and Knowsley AHA* (1999)

Employer's liability and indemnity insurance

An employer will be responsible for negligence against his own staff, or for negligence caused by his staff. The employer has responsibilities to make sure that there are in place:

- competent staff
- a safe place of work
- safe systems of work
- adequate staffing levels.

The reason this is important for the employer is because of the principle of vicarious liability. This is the principle that allows the employer to be sued for actions of an employee which may be negligent. The law of negligence requires that an employer should ensure the competency of its staff and should be able to take responsibility for negligent acts or omissions. Two conditions are needed for vicarious liability to apply:

- The person who was guilty of negligence must be an employee, so where the person who caused the accident was an independent contractor, the employer will not usually be liable.
- The act must be one for which the employer was responsible.

When a patient sues the employing hospital in negligence where injury has been caused by a nurse, it is always open to the patient to add the nurse as a second separate defendant, even where the principle of vicarious liability will mean that the employer is the main party being sued in negligence. In such cases the nurse will need separate legal representation and it is advisable for all nurses to ensure adequate protection against such an occurrence.

Most trade unions carry indemnity insurance as part of the services provided for the membership. This protects a nurse if a finding of negligence is made against the nurse and the indemnity insurance would meet the cost of compensation to be paid to the patient and the legal fees incurred.

The NMC recommends that all nurses consider the value of ensuring that indemnity insurance arrangements are in place. The NMC further advises that where there is no indemnity insurance in place, the nurse should notify each patient of this fact before providing treatment. The NMC does not require that indemnity insurance is a compulsory part of registration (NMC, 2002).

Summary

- An employer has duties to maintain a workplace to avoid claims of negligence.
- Vicarious liability means that the employer will be responsible for actions of his staff that cause negligence.

- A nurse can be added as a second defendant even where vicarious liability exists.
- The NMC recommends that nurses consider indemnity insurance.
- It is not a professional requirement to have indemnity insurance.

Activity

What professional organisation do you belong to? Check the membership booklet and read the section on indemnity insurance. Does it cover all the aspects of nursing practice that you are involved in? If not, contact your professional organisation in writing and check.

Contributory negligence and time limits

Contributory negligence is the defence that can reduce the amount of compensation to be paid. It applies where action on the part of the victim has contributed to the injury. The justification of a claim of contributory negligence is that the injury was at least in part the fault of the victim. The courts will have to assess the extent of that fault and then reduce the compensation by a percentage amount. For example, after a car accident a passenger may have compensation reduced by 25% if they were not wearing a seat belt. This is on the basis that the injuries would not have been so serious if the passenger had been wearing a seatbelt.

An action in negligence must be commenced within three years of the date of the accident. If an adult has an accident on 1 February 2006, the time limit will expire on 1 February 2009. If a child is injured, the law allows that child to reach adulthood of 18 years before starting the three years of the time limit. So if a child aged 6 years is injured, he will have until he reaches 21 years to bring his claim. It is for this reason that the records of children are kept for a much longer time than those of adults.

Where a person is injured but has no means of knowing this, the time limits start to run from the date that he discovered there was a problem. In the case of asbestos poisoning, for example, the individual may not realise he was affected until he has a later diagnosis. This may take place many years after the exposure.

Summary

- Contributory negligence can reduce the amount of compensation.
- The degree of reduction will depend on the degree of fault on the part of the victim.
- Time limits allow three years from the date of the injury for adults.
- Children have three years from the date of reaching the age of 18 to bring a claim.

Assault

There are four legal options of dealing with an assault at work.

Criminal actions against the assailant

The police will prosecute the assailant unless it is clear the assailant did not know what he or she was doing when carrying out the attack. Being attacked by a patient is never acceptable. Every assault should always be reported to the police. There is no breach of confidentiality as the nurse is reporting a crime. Most hearings into assault will take place in the magistrates' court and the nurse will need to attend as a witness. The magistrate has the power to imprison the assailant, and in some cases to make a limited award of compensation.

Suing the assailant

The nurse can bring proceedings in the County Court and claim compensation for physical and emotional injuries. If the nurse has lost time off work as a result of the attack, he or she can claim financial losses. Any claim must be made within three years of the date of the attack. All nurses should take legal advice in bringing this type of action. It is also important to know that the assailant has enough money to pay any compensation awarded.

Suing the employer

The employer has a duty to provide a safe system of work. If the nurse can prove the employer was negligent, he or she can claim compensation.

Applying to the CICA

The Criminal Injuries Compensation Authority (CICA) provides direct compensation to anyone who has been attacked. The mental state of the assailant is not important. The procedure is quicker, simpler and more private than the other three options. The nurse must make a claim within two years of the attack, and must prove that the attack happened and was reported to the police. The injuries suffered must meet a minimum value of £1000. Bruising or minor shock will not be sufficient to meet this limit.

Practical advice: what to do if you are attacked
- Complete an accident form as soon as possible.
- Contact the police and ask for a crime reference number.
- Ask other witnesses to write down what they saw.
- Report the attack to your manager.
- Make a report to Occupational Health.

- See your GP and make sure a record of the assault is in your medical records.
- Contact your professional organisation for assistance.

Application to accountability

Negligence is based on a series of principles which can be readily understood by nurses. This enables nurses to consider actions in the health care setting and assess whether any of the principles of negligence have been fulfilled. It is important to recognise that it is only where all the elements of the negligence case have been proved that a claim can be successful. Where this is the case, there are systems for calculating the amount of compensation to be paid.

The key issue to bear in mind is that the law does not judge the behaviour or action of the nurse by a moral standard when assessing whether she or he broke the standard of care. It is only if there are consequences that have a direct impact on the patient that the law becomes interested in assessing what the standard of care should have been.

This is a contrast to the way that the NMC will react to poor standards of care. The NMC Code of Conduct is based on the way that a nurse behaves, and breaking the Code of Conduct is not dependent on whether there were adverse consequences for the patient. The professional standards of the NMC focus on the standards of practice, whereas the law of negligence focuses on the consequences to the patient.

There have been calls to change the system of negligence in health care so that the patient can learn more easily what has happened and what steps are being put in place to make sure no similar injury is caused to another patient. The debate around this continues.

By now, you should be able to:

- avoid defensive nursing practice in relation to negligence
- be confident about the four principles of any negligence claim
- distinguish the standards of care required by law from those required by the NMC
- apply the law relating to negligence in the framework of accountability.

Summary

- A risk of negligence should not be used to justify defensive practice.
- The courts will require that causation exists before criticising a fall in the standard of care.
- The NMC does not need to know that causation exists in order to criticise a nurse for a fall in the standard of care.
- Debate continues around reform of the negligence system.

Useful website

Action Against Medical Accidents (an independent charity that promotes patient safety): www.avma.org
Law Society for England and Wales (has a useful section on clinical negligence): www.lawsociety.org.uk
Nursing and Midwifery Council: www.nmc-uk.org

References

Alcock v. *Chief Constable of South Yorkshire Police* [1991] 4 All ER 907.
Barnett v. *Chelsea and Kensington* [1968] 1 All ER 1068.
Bolam v. *Friern Barnet Management Committee* [1957] 2 All ER 118.
Bolitho v. *City and Hackney Health Authority* [1997] 4 All ER 771.
Briordy v. *St Helens and Knowsley AHA* [1999] Lloyds Rep Med 185.
Donoghue v. *Stephenson* [1932] AC 562.
Evans v. *Liverpool Corp* [1906] 1KB 160.
Nursing and Midwifery Council (2002) *Code of Professional Conduct*. NMC, London.
Occupier's Liability Act 1984. The Stationery Office, London.

Concepts: Consent

Learning objectives

This chapter is aimed at providing a clear and definitive context about consent for nurses. The aim of this chapter is to provide sufficient information for nurses to understand the principles of consent and how they are applied in particular health care situations.

The learning objectives for this chapter are to:

- set out why consent is important
- define consent
- describe the three principles of consent
- assess consent for children
- assess consent for adults
- assess consent for adults who cannot consent
- consider consent forms
- place the importance of consent in the context of accountability.

Introduction

Obtaining consent affirms the patient's right to self determination and autonomy. There is an ethical, professional and legal acknowledgment that a decision to consent to treatment involves a decision making process by the autonomous individual which will include that individual's values, circumstances, choices and attitude.

The changes which put the patient or client at the heart of the health service have led to a greater awareness of patients' rights. There is a greater responsibility on health care staff to respond to patients on an individual basis, taking into account the cultural, religious and personal preferences of the patient. The law of consent is based on an ethical approach to the value of autonomy, and reliance on the use of best interests when the individual lacks autonomy to provide consent.

The NMC Code of Professional Conduct has a separate section on consent (NMC, 2002). Clause 3 requires that 'as a registered nurse, midwife or health visitor, you must obtain consent before you give any treatment or care'. Figure 9.1 sets out clause 3 in full (see p. 129).

This professional duty recognises the value of autonomy in clause 3.2 and states that a refusal to receive treatment must be protected even where this may result in harm or death to the individual. The professional duty also requires that the nurse gives information that is accurate and truthful. It must be presented in such a way as to make it easily understood.

Summary

- Obtaining consent affirms the autonomy of the individual.
- Consent is recognised in ethical, professional and legal settings.
- The need to put the patient at the heart of health care raises the importance of consent.
- There is established law on consent which is based on tested ethical principles.
- These principles are endorsed in the NMC Code of Professional Conduct.

Why consent is important

Nurses must only carry out nursing care or treatment that involves physical contact with the patient's body after consent has been given. Without consent, the touching of the patient's body will not be lawful.

It is now an established part of law that no treatment may be given to an individual, whether it be clinical or nursing, unless the patient has consented to the treatment. If health professionals proceed with treatment without the patient's consent, they are vulnerable to an action in battery.

This could have two consequences. Firstly, the patient could sue the nurse or the employer for compensation, even if no harm occurred. For example, if a nurse gives an injection to patient without his or her consent, the administration will not be lawful and the nurse could be sued, even though the outcome was beneficial to the health of the patient. Second, the nurse could face a criminal prosecution. No prosecution has yet been brought against a nurse for failing to obtain consent but criminal investigations have been considered against some surgeons for failing to obtain consent.

The courts will protect the autonomy of the individual to make decisions about health care. In the celebrated American case nearly a century ago, *Schloendoff* v. *Society of New York Hospital* (1914), Cardozo J stated 'Every human being of adult years and sound mind has a right to determine what shall be done with his own body; and a surgeon who performs an operation without the patient's consent commits an assault'.

In the UK a more recent case echoed this principle. In *Airedale NHS Trust* v. *Bland* (1993), Lord Mustill underlined the respect the law gives to autonomy: 'If the patient is capable of making a decision whether to permit treatment and decides not to permit it his choice must be obeyed, even if on any objective view it is contrary to his best interests.'

Summary

- Touching another person must take place with their consent.
- If there is no consent, a battery has taken place.
- There are two legal consequences for a battery.
- A civil action can take place where the nurse is sued.
- A criminal action can take place where the nurse is prosecuted.
- This importance of autonomy is reflected in America as well as the UK.

Case study 9.1: Treatment without consent is unlawful even where the outcome is beneficial

The oldest case covering consent and the unlawful touching of a person was heard in America in 1905. This was a case of battery in relation to medical treatment. In this case, the patient gave his consent to surgery being carried out on his ear. Under anaesthetic, the surgeon discovered a disease far more prevalent in the opposite ear and proceeded to operate on that other ear.

After the surgery, the patient discovered that he had had surgery on both ears when he had only given his consent for treatment on one ear. He sued the surgeon and claimed this was a battery. He won. The court held that the doctor should have obtained the patient's consent before proceeding to operate on the other ear. This was in spite of an acknowledgement by all parties that the patient actually benefited from the operation, and that no physical harm took place.

The principle at issue was the violation of the patient's autonomy. The court agreed that he should know no treatment would take place unless he had given his consent.

Mohr v. *Williams* (1905)

'3.1 All patients and clients have a right to receive information about their condition. You must be sensitive to their needs and respect the wishes of those who refuse or are unable to receive information about their condition. Information should be accurate, truthful and presented in such a way as to make it easily understood. You may need to seek legal or professional advice, or guidance from your employer, in relation to the giving or withholding of consent.

3.2 You must respect patients' and clients' autonomy – their right to decide whether or not to undergo any health care intervention – even where a refusal may result in harm or death to themselves or a foetus, unless a court of law orders to the contrary. This right is protected in law, although in circumstances where the health of the foetus would be severely compromised by any refusal to give consent, it would be appropriate to discuss this matter fully within the team, and possibly to seek external advice and guidance.

3.3 When obtaining valid consent, you must be sure that it is:
– given by a legally competent person
– given voluntarily
– informed.

3.4 You should presume that every patient and client is legally competent unless otherwise assessed by a suitably qualified practitioner. A patient or client who is legally competent can understand and retain treatment information and can use it to make an informed choice.

3.5 Those who are legally competent may give consent in writing, orally or by cooperation. They may also refuse consent. You must ensure that all your discussions and associated decisions relating to obtaining consent are documented in the patient's or client's health care records.

3.6 When patients or clients are no longer legally competent and thus have lost the capacity to consent to or refuse treatment and care, you should try to find out whether they have previously indicated preferences in an advance statement. You must respect any refusal of treatment or care given when they were legally competent, provided that the decision is clearly applicable to the present circumstances and that there is no reason to believe that they have changed their minds. When such a statement is not available, the patients' or clients' wishes, if known, should be taken into account. If these wishes are not known, the criteria for treatment must be that it is in their best interests.

3.7 The principles of obtaining consent apply equally to those people who have a mental illness. Whilst you should be involved in their assessment, it will also be necessary to involve relevant people close to them; this may include a psychiatrist. When patients and clients are detained under statutory powers (mental health acts), you must ensure that you know the circumstances and safeguards needed for providing treatment and care without consent.

3.8 In emergencies where treatment is necessary to preserve life, you may provide care without patients' or clients' consent, if they are unable to give it, provided you can demonstrate that you are acting in their best interests.

3.9 No-one has the right to give consent on behalf of another competent adult. In relation to obtaining consent for a child, the involvement of those with parental responsibility in the consent procedure is usually necessary, but will depend on the age and understanding of the child. If the child is under the age of 16 in England and Wales, 12 in Scotland and 17 in Northern Ireland, you must be aware of legislation and local protocols relating to consent.

3.10 Usually the individual performing a procedure should be the person to obtain the patient's or client's consent. In certain circumstances, you may seek consent on behalf of colleagues if you have been specially trained for that specific area of practice.

3.11 You must ensure that the use of complementary or alternative therapies is safe and in the interests of patients and clients. This must be discussed with the team as part of the therapeutic process and the patient or client must consent to their use.'

Figure 9.1   NMC Code of Professional Conduct on consent.

The three principles of consent

Consent is the legal means by which the patient gives a valid authorisation for treatment or care. Consent is the permission given by a person to be touched by another. The legal principles match the professional principles of respect for autonomy for the individual. The legal basis of consent is therefore identical to the professional requirement that nurses need consent before carrying out any treatment. The case law on consent has established three principles, explained below, which must all be satisfied before any consent given by a patient can be sufficient. Once the three principles have been established, a valid consent has been given to treatment or care.

The first principle: consent should be given by someone with capacity

The person giving consent must have the capacity to do so. It is vital that a person giving consent has the capacity to understand what is involved in the proposed treatment. It is accepted that adults over the age of 16 have the relevant capacity to understand and make their own decisions about medical and nursing treatment.

Children and young adults under 16 do not lose an automatic right to give consent. The famous case of *Gillick* in 1985 looked at consent for young persons under the age of 16. The principle laid down in *Gillick* is that a competent child has the right to give consent to medical treatment. The consent issue arises when he or she is of sufficient understanding and intelligence to enable him or her to understand fully what is proposed.

Adults over 16 years who do not have the mental ability to make their own choices will not be able to consent to treatment or care. This cannot be given by another adult, so the Adults with Incapacity (Scotland) Act 2000 and the Mental Capacity Act 2005 in England and Wales set out the process to be used to provide healthcare to adults who cannot make their own decisions.

Summary

- A person must have the capacity to be able to give consent.
- Young persons below 16 years of age may have the capacity to give consent.
- The test for young persons under 16 years of age was decided in the *Gillick* case.
- The test is that the person must have the intelligence and understanding to understand what is involved.
- Adults who do not have the relevant capacity are not able to give consent.
- In that situation legislation sets out the process to decide whether the treatment is beneficial.

The second principle: sufficient information should be given to the patient

The patient or client must be able to give informed consent to the proposed treatment. The issue of informed consent has provoked much discussion among health professionals. Just how much information needs to be given to a patient before they have enough on which to make a decision? The legal cases over the years have decided that the following components are part of the information that should be given:

- material risks
- alternatives to the treatment
- the nature and consequences of the proposed treatment.

How does an individual nurse decide what information should be given and what can be held back? The test for this was formulated in the case of *Bolam* v. *Friern Barnet Management Committee* (1957), where the court decided that the standard of care required of a professional is to act in accordance with a recognised body of professional opinion and practice. In nursing, the standard is determined by the nursing profession itself and not by reference to a particular patient. This standard of care has been criticised for failing to give sufficient weight to the patient's own circumstances, and it has been suggested that a nurse or doctor should provide the patient with all the information in their possession in order to enable the patient to make an informed decision. This has been largely rejected by the courts as being impractical and overburdensome on the health professional.

Summary

- Information is the second part of a valid consent.
- The amount of information to be given to a patient has been considered by the courts.
- Information should include material risks, alternatives to the treatment and the nature and consequences of the proposed treatment.
- The standard of information will be decided by reference to the standard that exists for the profession.
- It is not necessary to tell the patient every aspect of information about the proposed treatment.

Case study 9.2: How much information is needed?

The most famous case on how much information should be given is *Sidaway* in 1985. Amy Sidaway agreed to an operation. She was not told that there was a very small risk that her spinal cord might be damaged. In the operation she suffered partial paralysis. She argued that she would not have consented to the

Continued

operation if she had been told of this risk. Her claim in court was that her whole consent was invalid as she had not received sufficient information to make an informed consent.

This argument was rejected by the House of Lords who found that the doctor had fulfilled his duties in relation to informed consent by telling her of the material risks, alternatives to the treatment and the nature and consequences of the proposed treatment. There is a duty on the doctor to assess whether the patient requires any further information. There is, however, no duty imposed by law on a health care professional to inform the patient of *all* the likely risks or advantages in the proposed treatment. The courts have held that the extent of what to tell the patient is within the doctor's discretion. If the patient asks questions, these should be answered truthfully, but again the doctor has discretion as to the amount of information that should be volunteered and he or she can withhold information for good reasons. This may require later justification if the case ever comes to court.

Sidaway v. *Board of Governors of Bethlem Royal Hospital* (1985)

The third principle: the consent must be freely given

Consent must be freely given. This means that no threats or implied threats must be used. Threats such as the use of a compulsory section under the Mental Health Act 1984 if treatment is not accepted would make the consent invalid. Whether treatment is voluntary will depend on what information is given to the patient and how this is presented. Coercion or manipulation of the patient would tend to imply that consent has not been obtained voluntarily.

In this situation, even where the patient signs a consent form the consent will be invalid because it was obtained in an unlawful manner. If a patient is told that he can have a drink when he is thirsty but only if he takes some medication beforehand, this may suggest that some form of coercion has been used by the nurse in the consent process for the medication. It may be arguable that the patient felt there was no real choice being given. If so, the medication has been given without consent.

Summary

- Consent must be freely given.
- There must be no coercion or undue influence.
- If the consent is not freely given, it becomes an unlawful consent.

Activity

Read clause 3 of the NMC Code of Professional Conduct. What do you think you would do if one of your patients refused treatment but you suspected this was because he or she was being pressured by an aggressive partner?

Case study 9.3: Undue influence

In a case in 1992, a woman known as Ms T, 22 years old, was involved in a car accident. While in hospital she told medical staff both orally and in writing that she did not want a blood transfusion should one become necessary. She was with her mother when she made these statements and her mother told staff that she was a committed Jehovah's Witness.

The woman's condition deteriorated and she was placed on a ventilator. When it became apparent that a blood transfusion would be required she was unable to give specific consent or refusal. She was given the blood transfusion. She survived and when she was well enough she took legal action against the hospital. She claimed that her autonomy had not been respected.

The Court of Appeal upheld the view that a competent adult patient has a right to refuse medical treatment even if the outcome will be that the patient will die. This has to be respected by the medical and nursing staff. In this case the court found that the influence by Ms T's mother was so significant that it was equivalent to duress. The court found that this undue influence made Ms T's refusal invalid. There was therefore no battery on the part of the doctor.

The Court of Appeal also considered the nature of the statements made by Ms T before she lost her capacity. The Court of Appeal stated that three criteria are needed for a valid advance refusal of treatment:

1. The patient must have capacity to consent or refuse the treatment at the time the refusal was made.
2. The patient must have anticipated and intended his decision to apply to the kind of situation that arose and the consequence of a refusal in that situation. This places the doctor under a duty to explain these matters to the patient so that she can make a valid decision to refuse treatment. Any attempt to mislead or misinform the patient would make a refusal invalid.
3. The patient's decision must be reached without undue influence.

Re T (1992)

Consent and young people

Giving consent

The law recognises that adults over 16 can make their own decisions about medical and nursing treatment, and legal provision is made for them to give consent for medical and nursing care in section 8 of the Family Law Reform Act 1969.

The more problematic area concerns adolescents below the age of 16. Children and young adults under 16 do not lose an automatic right to give consent. The famous case of *Gillick* in 1985 looked at consent for young persons under the age of 16. The House of Lords decided that it would be illogical to deny a young person under 16 any legal ability to consent by reference to his or her age alone. The House of Lords was aware that many young people under 16 have the intelligence and maturity to make clinical decisions on their own behalf, and it would be unreal to deny them the right to choose.

This judgement now allows young persons under 16 years to consent to treatment provided they have sufficient understanding and intelligence to enable them to understand fully what is proposed. The doctor or nurse proposing to carry out the treatment must be satisfied that the young person under 16 years of age has the maturity, intelligence and understanding to comprehend what is involved. If the doctor or nurse believes the young person has this mental and emotional ability, the child can consent despite being below 16 years.

The question of deciding whether the adolescent is capable of understanding is determined by the doctor, although it is likely that nurses, for example, would be able to give treatment to children where they make a professional assessment that the child has the understanding to know what is proposed and be involved in the nursing treatment.

This legal case has now been incorporated in legislation. It is in the Children Act 1989 for England and Wales. In Scotland, the Age of Legal Capacity (Scotland) Act 1991 gives authority in Scotland to young persons of sufficient understanding to consent to treatment.

Where the child is not capable of giving consent the guardian of a child under the age of 16 years may give valid consent on behalf of the child.

Summary

- Between 16 and 18 years, young persons have statutory authority to give consent.
- Adults over 18 are automatically assumed to have capacity.
- Young persons between 16 and 18 years have legal assumption about their capacity to give consent.
- Under 16 years, young people can give consent if they are Gillick competent.
- The test is whether the young person has sufficient understanding and intelligence to understand fully what is proposed.
- The assessment of capacity can be carried out by the health professional who proposes to carry out the treatment.
- Where a child does not have capacity to give consent, the consent can be given by a parent or guardian.

Refusing consent

The courts will allow a child to give consent but are more ambivalent about allowing a child to refuse consent, particularly where that may result in serious detriment to the child's health. Where a nurse is confronted with a strong difference of opinion between a child and a parent or guardian over proposed treatment, the nurse should always seek advice to ensure the correct weight is given to the child's wishes. In some situations it may be necessary to ask the court to decide between the conflicting wishes, where the consequences for the child in refusing the treatment would be significant for that child.

The Department of Health has published guidance on this aspect of consent with children, setting out how the law should be followed. This means that if the child is competent to give consent, she is to be regarded as competent to refuse consent. If the nurse or doctor is concerned about the consequences of a refusal for the child, the Department of Health gives guidance on when such cases should be taken to court (Department of Health, 2001).

Summary

- An ability to give consent does not automatically mean the young person can refuse consent.
- Parents or guardians in very rare cases can override the young person's refusal of consent.
- Nurses faced with a conflict between a young person and the parents should take legal advice.
- In some cases the courts will need to decide whether the young person's refusal can be supported.

Case study 9.4: Refusal of consent by a young person

The following case dealt with the situation where a young woman wanted to refuse treatment.

In *Re W* (1992) the Local Authority asked the court to grant them permission to use a nasogastric tube if this should become medically required on a 16-year-old girl with anorexia nervosa. The court found the girl was a Gillick competent child and of sufficient understanding to make an informed decision as to medical treatment. However the court held that she was not competent to refuse such treatment and they had little difficulty in overriding her refusal by assessing what would be in her best interests and ordering the appropriate treatment. The court could have assessed whether she had a mental illness in which case they would have been able to decide whether the treatment could have been authorised under the Mental Health Act 1983. By ensuring that the discussion remained focused on the autonomy of the individual girl, the court held true to the development of the earlier case law in this area.

Re W (1992)

Consent and adults

Adults who refuse treatment

The courts have consistently maintained the right to personal autonomy of an individual even where the outcome is that the patient may die. Any health care professional who ignores a valid refusal and carries out treatment will commit a battery. This means, for example, that a terminally ill patient can refuse to receive any further treatment and the doctor or nurse who accords with these wishes will not be held responsible for committing the crime of aiding and abetting a suicide. In fact, if the nurse does provide treatment against the patient's wishes, she will be vulnerable to a claim in battery. This is a further situation where ethical principles may clash, in this case autonomy and paternalism.

The right to refuse treatment may have some public policy limitations, particularly where the patient is refusing nursing care. There has not yet been a legal case where the patient refuses all forms of basic nursing care, so there are no clear guidelines at this stage. Professional guidance has been produced by the BMA on this issue (BMA, 1995). This guidance suggests that the court would probably not allow a refusal of nursing treatment to the extent that the individual is effectively left abandoned by society. It is likely that a patient could not validly refuse basic nursing care where public policy grounds were involved. This may include situations where the patient refuses to have treatment for pressure sores or to be cleaned, particularly where the patient is in an environment with others. Factors to be taken into account would include the interests of other health care professionals, or other patients who may be affected by a patient's refusal of basic nursing treatment.

Summary

- Adults can refuse medical treatment even where the consequence is that the patient may die.
- Health professionals have to respect this refusal of treatment.
- A failure to do so would mean that a battery has taken place.
- There may be public policy limitations on the extent to which a person can refuse basic nursing care.

Adults who cannot consent

Some adults do not have the capacity to provide consent to treatment or care. This may be most obvious in adults who suffer from a form of dementia. The complication with illnesses such as dementia is that the adult's capacity may vary depending on the severity of the illness on a particular day.

The adult suffering from dementia may have periods of complete lucidity where he or she can determine exactly what they wish in terms of medical or nursing care. On other occasions they may not. In these situations it will be necessary for the nurse to assess the patient's ability to understand the proposed treatment or care before each procedure takes place. Dementia may be a situation where medical technology will allow a more clear assessment of these periods of fluctuating capacity, but in the meantime it remains one of the hardest areas to resolve in terms of capacity and consent.

Some difficulty may exist for nurses who are motivated to act in the best interests of the patient. When the adult's choice accords with nursing practice the level of competence of that person, particularly if he or she has fluctuating capacity, is rarely assessed. Since the adult agrees with the treatment that is being proposed, many nurses automatically assume that the adult has capacity to consent. Because the treatment being proposed will always be in the patient's own interests, it is assumed that a patient who consents to that treatment is showing the necessary capacity to understand what is involved.

It seems that it may only be where the patient refuses treatment that an evaluation of capacity takes place. The importance of a refusal from an adult seems to be that it triggers a fresh evaluation of understanding, but it does not mean, because the person refuses to agree with the nurse's proposals, that he or she has necessarily lost the understanding that is crucial to give consent. There have been no cases dealing with this problem yet which would provide legal guidance.

In such a situation it seems that nurses demand a much higher level of understanding in order to satisfy themselves that the patient has capacity because he or she is now actively choosing a course not deemed to be in his or her best interests.

Summary

- Evaluation of capacity is the key to deciding whether a person has lost capacity on a temporary or a permanent basis.
- Adults who cannot consent can be treated in their best interests.
- The best interests of a patient include the whole assessment of their welfare.

Adults with mental illness

Adults who are incapable of giving consent because of mental illness can receive treatment under the provisions of the Mental Health Act 1983 for that disorder. However, there may be some situations where a person with a mental disorder may require medical treatment for some other condition. The Mental Capacity Act 2005 sets out the process to be used where this treatment is not connected to the mental illness. In such circumstances there will be a hearing before a judge to determine whether the proposed treatment is in that person's best interests.

It is important to be clear about the difference in providing treatment for the mental illness and for other health conditions. Where treatment is for a condition unrelated to the mental illness, the individual will have capacity if he can show:

- he understands the proposed treatment
- he believed what he had been told about it
- he was capable of balancing the risks.

Case study 9.5: Mental health and nonrelated health treatment

The court has held that patients with mental disorder can refuse treatment for a condition unrelated to that disorder.

In September 1993 doctors at Broadmoor Hospital discovered gangrene in a patient's foot and informed him that unless the foot and part of the leg were amputated he faced imminent death. The patient, who suffered from chronic paranoid schizophrenia, was transferred to the local hospital. He refused to consent to the amputation.

He applied to the court for an injunction restraining the hospital and the surgeons from amputating his leg both then and in the future unless he gave his express, written, valid consent. The judge was satisfied that the patient understood the proposed treatment, believed what he had been told about it and that the patient was capable of balancing the risks. Although his general capacity was impaired the judge found that it was not established that the patient did not understand the nature, purpose and effects of the treatment he refused.

The ruling in that case gives clear authority for the legal binding status of advance directives and this has importance particularly for mental health patients who may wish to give an advance directive about their future treatment. A patient who suffers from psychotic states of mind may have rational and lucid periods where he or she has sufficient capacity to make a decision on future mental, medical and nursing treatment.

Re C (1994)

Emergency treatment

What about the patient who is admitted in a state of unconsciousness and is clearly unable to provide consent to any proposed emergency treatment? It would be difficult to support a view that any subsequent touching or treatment would constitute battery in the absence of consent, because it is simply not possible to obtain this from the patient.

The law accepts that treatment should be given where it is in the best interests of the patient to save life or preserve health. In these circumstances there is no necessity to obtain consent.

This is not the same for non-urgent medical or nursing treatment. Where this needs to be given but is not necessary to save life or preserve life, it would be unlawful to proceed with that treatment. It is necessary in those situations to wait for the patient to regain consciousness and then obtain consent.

Summary

- The law of consent allows treatment to be given in emergency situations.
- Such treatment will not be regarded by the law as a battery.
- The emergency must be to save life or preserve health.
- Non-urgent treatment should wait for the patient's consent.

Consent forms

Consent can be given orally or by implied action. If a person who cannot speak sees that the nurse is about to take his temperature, he can open his mouth to receive the thermometer and this action can be regarded as implied consent.

Most hospitals require patients and clients to sign a consent form to agree to invasive treatment, and some health professionals have mistakenly placed too much emphasis on a signature being obtained on a form. A signed consent form does not prove that the consent is valid. It is usually good evidence that a discussion has taken place about consent. A consent form is important evidence although it should never be the only factor taken into account in establishing that full and proper consent has been obtained.

Summary

- Consent forms are confirmation that the discussion on consent has taken place.
- A consent form is not the most important part of the consent process.
- Questions that the patient has raised can be recorded on the consent form.
- A signed consent form is good evidence that a discussion on consent has taken place.

Conclusion

By now, you should be able to:
- understand the critical importance of consent in health care
- be confident about how a person can consent to treatment
- be confident about when a person can refuse consent
- assess the importance of consent forms in nursing practice.

Useful websites

British Medical Council: www.bma.org.uk
Department of Health: www.dh.gov.uk This website has a section on current guidance on consent. Type 'consent' in the main search engine which will show the range of current documents giving guidance and advice.

References

Adults with Incapacity (Scotland) Act 2000. The Stationery Office, London.
Age of Legal Capacity (Scotland) Act 1991. The Stationery Office, London.
Airedale NHS Trust v. *Bland* [1993] AC 789.
British Medical Association (1995) *Advance statements about medical treatment.* BMA, London.
Bolam v. *Friern Barnet Management Committee* [1957] 2 All ER 118.
Children Act 1989. The Stationery Office, London.
Department of Health (2001) *Seeking consent; working with children.* DoH, London.
Family Law Reform Act 1969. The Stationery Office, London.
Gillick v. *West Norfolk and Wisbech Area Health Authority* [1985] 3 All ER 402.
Mental Capacity Act 2005. The Stationery Office, London.
Mental Health Act 1983. The Stationery Office, London.
Mohr v. *Williams* (1905) 104 NW 12.
Nursing and Midwifery Council (2002) *Code of Professional Conduct.* NMC, London.
Re C [1994] 1 All ER 819.
Re T [1992] 4 All ER 649.
Re W [1992] 4 All ER 627.
Schloendoff v. *Society of New York Hospital* (1914) 211 NY 125.
Sidaway v. *Board of Governors of Bethlem Royal Hospital* [1985] 1 All ER 643.

Applications: Confidentiality

Learning objectives

This chapter will consider the relationship of privacy, trust and sharing of information between a patient and a nurse. Confidentiality is an important part of the nurse–patient relationship, and this chapter will show how it can be applied in each area of accountability that has already been described, to show the four pillars of accountability in practice.

The learning objectives for this chapter are to:

- understand the importance of trust in relation to confidence
- be clear about the legal sources of confidentiality
- clarify the extent of professional obligations in confidence
- critically evaluate the ethical issues in confidentiality
- understand the role of the employer in relation to confidence
- be clear about data protection and record keeping
- apply the four pillars of accountability in confidentiality.

Introduction

Confidentiality is a fundamental part of the clinical relationship. Any information given to a nurse by a patient should not be passed on to anyone outside the health care team without consent. The fundamental importance of trust between a health professional and the patient brings with it a duty of confidence. It is critical to the continuing trust in clinical relationships that information is treated with respect and is protected from disclosure unless the patient gives his or her consent.

It is important to distinguish between ownership of the health record and ownership of the information contained on the record. They are treated in different ways. The paper or computer hard drive on which records are created does not belong to the patient. It belongs to the GP or NHS Trust or health provider. As a result, the patient cannot ask to keep these records. However, the information that is contained on the record can be disclosed to the patient and in some situations must be disclosed to the patient.

In the past, patient records were kept secret even from patients and disclosure was generally only allowed with a court order. It is only since the late 1990s that legislation has been introduced to give patients rights of access to the health information about them. This is viewed as increasing patient autonomy and reducing medical paternalism.

The NMC Code of Professional Conduct (NMC, 2002) requires nurses to respect confidentiality and to ensure that information obtained in a relationship of trust is kept private unless consent has been given for this to be disclosed. Breaking the duty of confidence could lead to the nurse being referred to the NMC for investigation into fitness to practice.

The common law (made by judges) gives rights to individuals who believe that this duty to protect information has been broken. These rights can be used against the nurse on a personal basis or they can be used against the health provider. There is also a range of legislation that sets out the way that health information must be disclosed, how health records must be recorded and how information must be stored. (For a further discussion on the differences between common law and legislation, see Chapter 4.)

Summary

- The duty of trust is at the heart of the concept of confidentiality.
- The protection of trust is why confidential information must be protected.
- Protection for health information is given by law and by professional bodies.
- Ethical concerns and employment rights of privacy are applicable to confidentiality.
- Where confidentiality has been broken there are legal processes that allow patients to take action against the individual nurse or the health provider.
- The health record belongs to the NHS or health provider and not to the patient.
- The patient has rights to access the information on the health record.

Legal accountability

Common law: general principles

The nurse must keep in confidence all information received from a patient. Legal sanctions can be used against nurses who do not follow this basic legal principle. There have been no legal cases which deal with a nurse's breach of confidentiality but there has been one significant case involving a doctor, set out in Case study 10.1.

The common law principles are:

- Confidentiality is a fundamental part of the clinical relationship.
- Any information given to a nurse by a patient should not be passed on to anyone outside the health care team without consent.
- A breach of confidentiality can lead to a civil action.
- The remedy for a breach of confidentiality is a payment of compensation.
- This payment will have to be made personally by the nurse.
- A planned breach of confidentiality can be dealt with by an injunction hearing.
- An injunction will prevent the information being passed to a third party.
- A defence is that the breach of confidentiality was in the public interest.
- It is for the person who broke the confidence to prove that the breach of confidence was justified in the public interest.
- The court will decide whether the public interest defence is justified.

Common law: making a disclosure to others

Because the main principle is that information must be protected, there are limited circumstances in which information can be disclosed outside the clinical relationship. The main reasons for making a disclosure to another person will take place in the following circumstances.

The patient has given his or her consent

Where the patient agrees that health information can be given to anyone, including members of his or her family, the nurse can disclose this information. If this permission has not been given, the nurse cannot give any health information to anyone including members of the family. This is the key justification for disclosure of information.

A court order requires the disclosure of the information

In a court case it may be necessary to have access to the health information of an individual. The solicitor will request disclosure of the information by sending a written form of consent to the patient. Where there is no consent, the solicitor can apply to the court for an order making the disclosure. The health organisation receiving this court order is required to follow the terms of the order. Failure to do so may be a contempt of court. Nurses are under a legal duty to comply with the terms of the court order, and no breach of confidentiality occurs in these circumstances. Any nurse receiving a letter from a solicitor asking for health information must be sure that there is consent from the patient for this disclosure.

There is legislation that requires the information to be disclosed

There are some situations where central notification of a particular type of treatment or prevalence of a specified disease is required by legislation. Examples of this include central notification of abortion, which must include the name and address of the woman. This information must be given to the Chief Medical Officer (Abortion Regulations, 1991). Other examples include notifiable diseases such as dysentery, diphtheria, or gastroenteritis as well as food poisoning, where disclosure is a requirement of the Public Health Act 1984.

The nurse considers it in the public interest to make the disclosure

The nurse may make a disclosure if she or he considers that it would be in the public interest to do so. There may be circumstances where the information received by the nurse is so significant that she or he wants to make this known to someone else. For example, if a child informs the nurse that she is involved in drug trafficking the nurse may want to pass this information to the police. It is critical for the nurse to understand that in law there is no *duty* on the nurse to make this disclosure, but there is a *discretion* that allows the nurse to make this disclosure. This means that the law does not require that the nurse *must* make a disclosure but it allows that she *may* make this disclosure. Whenever the nurse believes that this public interest exists, it is always preferable to secure the patient's consent to disclosure of the information.

Summary

- There is a legal duty to keep information confidential.
- There are four ways in which information can disclosed.
- The most common ground for disclosure is with the patient's consent.
- A court order overrides the patient's confidentiality.
- There may be legislation that requires disclosure of information.
- The nurse may feel that disclosure is required in the public interest.
- There is no legal duty to make a disclosure in the public interest.

Case study 10.1: Common law of confidence

The key English case on this subject is *W* v. *Egdell* where a prisoner in a secure hospital requested a review so that he could transfer to a regional secure unit. Dr Egdell, an independent psychiatrist, prepared a report which stated that the patient was not safe to be transferred. A very short time later the patient was due for a routine review of his detention and Dr Egdell was concerned that his report would not be included in the review. He sent a copy of his report to the Medical Director of the Hospital and the Home Office.

The patient sued Dr Egdell for breach of confidence. The patient argued that the report should only be disclosed with his consent, and that he had not given this. The court held that a breach of confidence had taken place because Dr Egdell had not obtained consent from the patient.

Dr Egdell argued that disclosure was justified in the public interest, as the patient represented a risk of threat to society if he were to be discharged from the hospital. The Court of Appeal accepted this argument that the disclosure was justified because a real risk to public safety existed. However, the Court of Appeal said that only the most compelling circumstances could justify a doctor acting in this way. In every case the doctor should seek to obtain the patient's consent before breaching confidentiality.

W v. *Egdell* (1990)

Common law: consequences of breaking a confidence

The legal consequences of making an unauthorised disclosure are serious for the nurse. She can be sued for breach of confidence and she may be asked to pay compensation to the patient if the court finds that none of the grounds set out above have been satisfied. Vicarious liability will not apply in these circumstances as the nurse will not be acting under the duty of an employer. The nurse will be sued as an individual.

If there has been no consent for the disclosure of the information, the nurse may argue that disclosure was in the public interest. The court will have to decide whether it agrees with the nurse. There is a risk that this may not happen. If the court cannot find that there was a public interest defence, then a breach of confidence will be found and the nurse will be ordered to pay compensation.

If a person believes that information is about to be given to a third party, or perhaps given to the media, it is possible to go to court to ask for an injunction before the publication takes place. The person will ask the court for an order to prevent the publication taking place, on the grounds that it is breaking confidentiality.

Summary

- A nurse can be sued as an individual if she makes a breach of confidence.
- Compensation can be ordered by the court for a breach of confidence.
- The patient can also ask for an injunction to prevent a breach of confidence.

Legislation

Legislation has been passed by Parliament that allows the patient to have access to the information in specified circumstances, as follows.

Supreme Court Act 1981

Disclosure of health care information can be ordered by the court where it is needed for litigation. If a person is being sued by someone they suspect may have an illness or medical history that is relevant to the case, that person can ask the court for disclosure of that health information. A court order will override any attempt made by the other person to forbid disclosure of their health information. In most cases the court will ask what attempts have been made to obtain consent from the patient.

Access to Medical Reports Act 1988

This Act applies to reports made for insurance or employment purposes. The Act is limited in that it only covers medical reports from a doctor with responsibility for the clinical care of the individual. The individual must give consent for the doctor to provide a report directly to the insurance company. A copy of the report can be sent to the individual and, where disagreements arise, the individual is allowed to make comments on the report. A patient has a right to see a medical report compiled by a doctor with responsibility for his clinical care if this is then to be sent to an insurance company or employer.

Access to Health Records Act 1990

This provides a right of access by patients to their own manually-kept records created from 1 November 1991. Although the name of the Act suggests a move towards patient-controlled access to their records, the main power remains with the holder who can determine the individual's right of access. Most of the legal rights in this Act are now covered by the Data Protection Act 1998.

Data Protection Act 1998

This Act applies to electronically and manually stored data. It gives patients a right to see both computer and manual health records. A patient can have access to health information by giving sufficient notice in a required form. A request can be made in writing with payment of a fee plus reasonable photocopying charges. No fee can be charged for records which are less than 40 days old. Children who are capable of understanding the nature of such an application can request access. In some circumstances, parents can apply for access to their child's data.

The Act defines two types of individual: the data user (the person entering the information on the system) and the subject of that information. The Act covers health information which is defined as 'sensitive personal data'. The Act sets out principles that have to be followed by those using such information, and these principles apply to nurses.

It is open to the holder of the manually or electronically stored records to refuse disclosure if, in the opinion of the holder, that disclosure would cause serious harm to the physical or mental health of the patient. The Act does not require the holder of information to justify such a decision.

Summary

- Different Acts of Parliament provide different rights of access to health information.
- It is possible to deny a patient access to their records if it would cause serious harm to the patient or to another person.

Professional accountability

NMC Code of Professional Conduct

Anyone can make a complaint to the NMC about a breach of confidence. The NMC will deal with this through the fitness to practice system and may make an order for a caution or a striking off of the nurse. This may be in addition to any legal penalty that is imposed if the nurse is sued by the patient. The NMC Code of Professional Conduct, clause 5, deals with the professional duty of confidentiality. This is set out in Figure 10.1. It means that where a complaint is made by a patient to the NMC about a nurse, there are clearly defined principles against which the NMC can assess the behaviour of the nurse.

The professional standard set by the NMC follows the legal standards, and the NMC would expect disclosure of health information to take place according to the legal grounds. What is interesting about this clause in the Code of Conduct is that the NMC has attempted to set out a broad definition of what might be counted as within the parameters of best interest that may justify a professional disclosure. The NMC says this may be justified 'where disclosure is essential to protect the patient or client or someone else from the risk of significant harm'. This definition suggests that the interests of society take precedence over the individual's right to confidentiality where there is an indica-

As a registered nurse, midwife or health visitor, you must protect confidential information

5.1 You must treat information about patients and clients as confidential and use it only for the purposes for which it was given. As it is impractical to obtain consent every time you need to share information with others, you should ensure that patients and clients understand that some information may be made available to other members of the team involved in the delivery of care. You must guard against breaches of confidentiality by protecting information from improper disclosure at all times.
5.2 You should seek patients' and clients' wishes regarding the sharing of information with their family and others. When a patient or client is considered incapable of giving permission, you should consult relevant colleagues.
5.3 If you are required to disclose outside the team information that will have personal consequences for patients or clients, you must obtain their consent. If the patient or client withholds consent, or if consent cannot be obtained for whatever reason, disclosures may be made only where: – they can be justified in the public interest (usually where disclosure is essential to protect the patient or client or someone else from the risk of significant harm) – they are required by law or by order of a court.
5.4 Where there is an issue of child protection, you must act at all times in accordance with national and local policies.

Figure 10.1   NMC Code of Professional Conduct clause 5.

tion that people could be placed at *significant harm* without the disclosure of that information.

The NMC also confirms that it is the individual nurse's responsibility to justify a breach of confidentiality, and this responsibility cannot be delegated to another person. The NMC advises that where a breach of confidentiality has taken place, the nurse should keep a separate record of the reasons for this.

Summary

- The NMC gives specific guidance on confidentiality in clause 5 of the Code of Professional Conduct.
- The guidance is similar to the legal framework of accountability.
- The NMC has given guidance on what may define a professional public interest disclosure.
- The NMC reinforces that breaking confidence is a personal matter for the nurse.

Other professions' obligations

Other professional bodies may give wider guidance on confidentiality. The General Medical Council, for example, gives detailed guidance for doctors that may also be useful for nurses (GMC, 2000). Where nurses work in a multidisciplinary team and an issue of confidentiality arises, it will be important to check what professional guidance applies to each member of the team.

Summary

- Professional obligations will apply to each member of the health care team.
- Where an issue of confidentiality arises, each member should check the guidance from their own professional body.

Health care standards

Central guidance from different Government departments sets out ways in which health professionals are required to keep health information confidential. The Department of Health set out guidance on the law, ethics and employment standards in 1996 (Department of Health, 1996).

Caldicott Guardians are senior clinicians appointed by NHS Trusts to oversee the protection of confidential information (Department of Health, 1999a).

Further guidance from the Department of Health has been given on the length of time that records have to be stored (Department of Health, 1999b).

The Information Commission has been set up to provide a monitoring and advice service for those involved in processing computer records and in providing access under the Freedom of Information Act 2000. Guidance has been issued for those using health data (Information Commissioner, 2002).

Summary

- It is always important to check what national guidance has been published, to assess what practical information this contains.
- National standards may come from different Government departments or agencies.

Case study 10.2: Confidentiality in audit research tested in court

A case assessed whether the use of anonymised information for audit purposes was a breach of patient confidentiality. It was argued that there would be no mechanism to find out whether a patient had or had not given consent for the use of information for these purposes.

The Court of Appeal found that there was no breach of confidentiality as the information was only given to the company carrying out the audit in such a form that it would be impossible to identify the patient from the information

Continued

given. Because it was impossible to identify the patient, there was no breach of privacy between the treating clinician and the patient. The court said this would be the case even where it went against the patient's wishes.

R v. Department of Health ex parte Source Informatics Ltd. (2000)

Ethical accountability

Duty or discretion

There is no absolute duty to disclose information to a third party even where it would appear the patient is at risk. There is discretion on the nurse to do so. If the nurse does disclose this information, he or she should be aware of the potential need to justify their actions at a later date.

The dignity of the patient is a fundamental value at the heart of the relationship between the nurse and the patient. This means that however vulnerable the patient is, the nurse will work towards promoting and making sure that others respect the dignity of the individual. This involves making sure that privacy is provided for the patient, even if the patient does not appear to be concerned about this. It also means that the nurse will be careful to ensure that records are kept that are respectful about the patient, and that information that is shared among other health care professionals promotes the dignity of the patient.

Activity

Peter is a community psychiatric nurse. One of his clients, Janet, tells him that she has morbid thoughts about breaking into a nearby school to attack any member of staff who reminds her of an old teacher. Peter considers what steps he can take. What would you suggest are the actions he could take?

Commentary
This information relates to a broad group of people and there is no named third party. The issue is whether it is in the public interest for Peter to inform the head teacher of the potential threat and identify Janet to any or all of the teaching staff. There is no duty on Peter to inform the school about this, but a discretion is given to him by the law and by the NMC Code of Professional Conduct.

The first step is for Peter to try and obtain permission from Janet to take this information to the clinical team for further advice about the extent of the risk. He can then also consider whether the type of harm that is being discussed falls within the NMC Code. If it does, this will give him protection from fitness to practice proceedings if he uses his professional discretion to make the disclosure to the head teacher at the school or to the police.

He should make sure that he has taken legal advice from his professional body before taking either step as there is a risk that Janet may sue him for a breach of confidence. He should also make sure that he notifies Janet of what he is intending to do, so that he continues to be honest in the clinical relationship with her.

Public interest

Public interest covers the rights of wider society to be given information that may have a wide impact on society. When the first test-tube baby, Louise Brown, was born, the public interest in the development of the science may have justified the disclosure of her identity on public interest grounds. It is important for the nurse to understand that there is a difference between what is interesting the public and what is in the public interest. If a major Hollywood star is admitted to hospital with a stomach ulcer, this may be interesting to the public but a disclosure of this health information would most certainly not be in the public interest. However, if that Hollywood star had come from a country with a contagious disease, it may be in the public interest to warn others who had flown in from that country to seek medical attention.

Case study 10.3: Ethical issues around public interest

A journalist discovered doctors working in a hospital had contracted HIV and were diagnosed with AIDS. The journalist informed the hospital that publication would take place shortly, disclosing the names of the doctors. The hospital sought an injunction to prevent publication. The case went to court to consider whether the planned publication would be a breach of confidence. A further issue raised in the court case was whether the disclosure would be justified in the public interest.

The court found that the information about the doctors was confidential, and that it required a protection. When considering the issue of public interest, the court decided that proposed publication was not justified in the public interest, and granted an injunction to prevent this taking place. In order to give further protection, the court ordered that the names of the individuals should not appear in the court judgment.

X v. *Y* (1988)

Human rights

Article 8 of the European Convention on Human Rights gives each citizen a right to respect for private and family life. The right of confidentiality in Article 8 is not absolute, but has been considered in relation to protecting health information.

Summary

- The nurse must know the difference between a duty and a discretion in disclosing information.
- There is a difference between what is interesting to the public and the public interest.
- Wider society rights may justify a disclosure in the public interest.
- A nurse considering giving information to another person without consent should obtain professional or legal guidance.

Case study 10.4: Human rights and access to personal records

The 1990 Access to Health Records Act came into existence following a case heard in the European Court of Human Rights in 1990 in which the applicant claimed that the refusal by his local authority to provide him with information of records on his care was in breach of his right to respect for his private and family life under Article 8 of the Convention.

Gaskin v. *United Kingdom* (1990)

Case study 10.5: Human rights and access to medical records of a third party

In a case dealing with disclosure of medical records, a man was convicted of attempted manslaughter after failing to declare his HIV status to a number of sexual partners. At the trial an order was made that his wife's medical records be disclosed. These records were referred to, along with the wife's identity, in the judgment. She went to the European Court of Human Rights and claimed that her rights under Article 8 had been violated.

The court found that it had been necessary for her records to be used in the trial as this was both 'necessary in a democratic society' and proportionate. However, the disclosure of her identity was an infringement of her rights and she was awarded compensation. The requirement that the doctor give this evidence was not a violation, but where the identity of the patient was revealed that was a violation.

Z v. *Finland* (1998)

Employment accountability

There may be many situations at work where there is confusion about who may receive information from another person in relation to health matters. With the increase in multi-disciplinary team working, it is even more important to be clear about who can receive information from the nurse. This section considers the rights of different individuals to receive information from the nurse.

Other members of the health team

There is an implied presumption in law (echoed in the NMC Code of Conduct) that a patient has given implied consent for details about his health to be passed to members of the health care team. This has been described as the 'need to know' principle. It may be useful to consider whether a factsheet can be given to a patient where health records would be shared with many other health departments. This would include access for clerical staff who are sending papers or X-rays, as well as the treating staff.

Police

There is no legal or professional duty for a nurse or a doctor to answer any questions raised by the police about someone who may be a patient. There is equally no duty to provide access to medical records. Either course of action may be a breach of the legal or professional requirement to protect confidentiality. Where the police have a court order by way of a search warrant, this will specify the extent of information that can be disclosed.

Legislation provides that the nurse must disclose information to the police in connection with terrorism (Prevention of Terrorism (Temporary Provisions) Act 1989). It is always advisable to have a local policy that deals with the potential questioning of a patient by the police. Where the nurse is not sure, she should ask the police to wait until she takes advice from her employer or professional organisation.

Social services

Co-operation between health and social services may be particularly relevant in child protection. The Children Act 1989 sets out a duty for health authorities to co-operate with local authorities in relation to children, but the duty of confidence is protected even in this legislation, allowing the health authority to retain confidential information if would unduly prejudice its work. There is therefore no statutory duty to disclose information about suspected child abuse but there is a discretion that applies to all health staff, and the NMC may count this as being within its definition of public interest.

Solicitors

Where solicitors seek information about the health of their client or of another person, this should only be given where there is a signed consent form from that person, or a court order. If a case is heard in court a subpoena may be issued. This is an order requiring a person to attend court with the original records.

Family and friends

Family members may demand information on their relative, particularly if that person is in hospital. Very often this will take the form of a telephone request. The nurse should ensure that there is clear consent on the patient's notes about the identity of the person to whom information can and cannot be given. Failure to do so may mean that a breach of confidence has taken place.

Activity

You learn that Joe is HIV positive. He expressly forbids this information to be passed to his partner. You know that a risk of infection exists. How would you persuade Joe to give you permission to inform his partner? Consider how you would assess your responsibilities under the four pillars of accountability.

Occupational health

When a nurse visits the occupational health department as a patient, the information given to the occupational health nurse or doctor remains protected and should not be disclosed without consent. It is possible for the occupational health nurse to send a report to the employing manager, but this can only contain information that is disclosed with the consent of the nurse being treated.

Summary

- There may be different employment situations that affect confidentiality.
- Nurses need to be aware of the different distinctions in these relationships.

Practical tips for protecting confidentiality in clinical relationships

- Obtain consent wherever possible for disclosure to a third party.
- Consider telling the patient at the outset of a consultation that some information may be important to third parties and preferable to disclose. Discuss these issues with the patient so that he or she is aware of the nurse's own responsibilities in this matter.

- Discuss with other members of the health team and draw up an agreed contract of confidentiality so that patients are aware in advance where health information will be protected, and the possible circumstances where it may not.
- Document fully in writing where you feel a disclosure needs to take place and the patient refuses to give consent for this disclosure. This may be vital in any subsequent court proceedings where the defence of public interest is being relied upon.
- In *any* situations of doubt or worry, contact your professional organisation for guidance and legal advice where appropriate. Make a note of who you speak to, the date of the conversation and a summary of the advice you were given.

Activity

Alice is a world famous Hollywood actress and dancer. She was touring in London and damaged her knee. She is being treated in your hospital. The media know she is being treated on your ward. Draft a press statement that you would want Alice to approve, giving health information for disclosure to the waiting journalists.

Conclusion

By now, you should be able to:
- understand the process of applying the four pillars of accountability in confidentiality
- identify the elements of privacy, trust and sharing of information in health relationships
- take active steps in nursing practice to ensure that accountability in confidentiality is maintained.

Useful websites

Nursing and Midwifery Council: www.nmc-uk.org
Information Commission: www.dataprotection.gov.uk
General Medical Council: www.gmc-uk.org
Department of Health: www.dh.gov.uk

References

Abortion Regulations 1991, SI 1991, No 499. The Stationery Office, London.
Access to Health Records Act 1990. The Stationery Office, London.
Access to Medical Reports Act 1988. The Stationery Office, London.

Children Act 1989. The Stationery Office, London.

Data Protection Act 1998. The Stationery Office, London.

Department of Health (1996) *The Protection and Use of Patient Information: Guidance from the Department of Health*. DoH, London.

Department of Health (1999a) *Caldicott Guardians*. Health Service Circular 99/012. DoH, London.

Department of Health (1999b) *For the Record, managing records in the NHS Trusts and Health Authorities*. Health Service Circular 1999/053. DoH, London.

European Convention for the Protection of Human Rights and Fundamental Freedoms (1950). Council of Europe, Strasbourg.

Gaskin v. *United Kingdom* (1990) 21 EHRR 36.

General Medical Council (2000) *Confidentiality: protecting and providing information* GMC, London.

Information Commissioner (2002) *Use and Disclosure of Health Data; Guidance on the application of the Data Protection Act 1998*. Information Commissioner, London.

Nursing and Midwifery Council (2002) *Code of Professional Conduct*. NMC, London.

Prevention of Terrorism (Temporary Provisions) Act 1989. The Stationery Office, London.

Public Health Act 1984, section 11. The Stationery Office, London.

R v. *Department of Health ex parte Source Informatics Ltd* [2000] 1 All ER 786.

Supreme Court Act 1981. The Stationery Office, London.

W v. *Egdell* [1990] 1 All ER 835.

X v. *Y* [1988] 2 All ER 649.

Z v. *Finland* (1998) 25 EHRR 371.

Further Applications in Accountability

Learning objectives

This chapter sets out a range of different issues in nursing practice and applies the four pillars of accountability to each issue. This will enable you to see how the application of accountability in practice can be used to assess the issues in nursing practice. The examples have been chosen deliberately because of their complexity. This is to show you that the four pillars of accountability can be used in the most sensitive situations in nursing practice.

The learning objectives for this chapter are to:

- consider two areas of nursing practice: conscientious objection in abortion, and gift giving in palliative care
- apply the four pillars of accountability to any nursing situation
- understand the range of issues that can be considered in the framework of accountability
- be confident in your nursing practice using the framework of accountability.

Introduction

This chapter considers two applications in accountability

- conscientious objection in abortion
- gift giving in palliative care.

Each of these areas will be considered under the four pillars of accountability:

- professional
- ethical
- legal
- employment.

This will demonstrate the process of accountability in nursing practice. These examples have been chosen to highlight areas in nursing practice in which there are strong differences of view. The ethics of abortion are profound. Similarly, the reaction to termination has been a matter of conscientious objection of such importance that this is now recognised in legislation which carries over to employment practice. This range of reactions is recognised by professional guidance which accepts that there will be matters of individual conscience that have to be reconciled with the need to ensure that nursing practice is safe and competent.

The professional structures dealing with the withdrawal of treatment are based on a consideration of the needs of the individual and the protection given to that individual in their best interests. The issue of gifts as a complexity in this relationship is also considered.

Summary

- Even sensitive areas of nursing practice can be considered in an assessment of accountability.
- The following examples will show the application of accountability in practice.
- There are complex issues to be addressed in each issue.

Abortion and conscientious objection

The nurse who is working with people in the range of pre-life care advice and treatment may be engaged in a whole range of different specialist areas of practice. She may assist women and men in fertility treatment. She may provide advice on contraception for men and women. She may work with women seeking a termination of pregnancy. She may work with women who want to act as surrogate mothers. She may work with young people in providing sexual health education in an effort to reduce the incidence of teenage pregnancy. These are now specialist areas of nursing practice. This section considers only one of these areas: abortion. Because this is a wide ranging area of nursing practice, consideration is given to one aspect: conscientious objection. This is where a nurse wants to opt out of providing treatment or care for this type of procedure.

Scenario

Patricia is a newly qualified nurse working full time in the community and working for an agency every Saturday daytime. She never knows where the agency will send her to work. One Saturday she is asked to work at the local hospital. When she arrives she finds that the hospital is running additional clinics for women who want a termination. Patricia is very uneasy about staying on this ward as she has personal views on termination.

She tells the ward sister that she has difficulty in working this shift and makes a phone call to the agency urgently to see what they suggest. While she is waiting to be put through, she has to assess her accountability. The issues she will need to address are set out below under each pillar of accountability, followed by a commentary on the scenario.

Professional accountability

In the professional role of accountability, the nurse needs to be aware that the NMC Code of Professional Conduct (NMC, 2002) allows for conscientious objection but does not limit this to a particular area of practice. Clause 2.5 states: 'You must report to a relevant person or authority, at the earliest possible time, any conscientious objection that may be relevant to your professional practice. You must continue to provide care to the best of your ability until alternative arrangements are implemented.'

This means that while the NMC will allow conscientious objection, it can only apply when the nurse is sure that the care of the individual is not compromised and that alternative arrangements are in place.

Guidance about the professional approaches to take in relation to abortion was published by the Royal College of Obstetricians and Gynaecologists in 2004 in relation to requests for late induced abortion as well as patient information (RCOG, 2004).

The Department of Health has a wide range of publications on abortion, that includes policy and guidance and frequently asked questions on its website. This information is included as part of the overall section on sexual health. The House of Commons has also considered the professional issues linked to conscientious objection, arising from the legislation and its impact on healthcare professionals (HCSSC, 1989–90).

Activity

Read the patient information about abortion on the RCOG website at www.rcog.org.uk and compare this with the frequently asked questions on the Department of Health website at www.dh.gov.uk. Do you consider that the information given is adequate?

Ethical accountability

The division of opinion about the rights and responsibilities in pre-life situations can be extreme. This section considers three areas of ethical debate:

- the moral status of the foetus
- the maternal–foetal conflict
- conscientious objection.

Much of the ethical debate starts with a review of the moral status of the unborn child. It is quite common for those with particular religious beliefs to hold a view that all life is sacred and that the sanctity of life must be preserved. Others who have a grounding in a rights-based view of ethics will argue that the woman has complete autonomy over the control of her own body, and that this allows her to terminate a pregnancy. A newer form of moral debate now includes whether the father of the foetus has any rights to intervene to prevent the termination because of rights that should be given to the father.

Further ethical debate takes place over the balance of rights between the mother and the unborn child. Should the rights of the mother to decide whether or not to have treatment take greater precedence than the moral rights of the foetus? This is known as the maternal–foetal conflict, and is a conflict because of the difficulty in according one set of rights to either the mother or the foetus without infringing the rights of the other.

Conscientious objection is a third area of ethical debate. Where a health care professional does not want to take part in a termination of pregnancy, the ethical values of society recognise that this may be a situation where a clinical professional would want to withdraw from providing care. This ethical right reinforces the ethical values of autonomy of the individual nurse.

There may be situations where the nurse has the skills and expertise to carry out a particular procedure but does not want to become involved because of ethical issues that are personal to the nurse. The most common situations where this occurs are in relation to abortion. There may be other situations where the nurse wants to exercise conscientious objection because of the nature of the outcome of the procedure, for example research on young children who are not able to provide their own permission. It is important for the nurse to be aware of her own values so that she is clear about where she would have a conscientious objection to an aspect of nursing care.

Case study 11.1: Father's rights in preventing an abortion

Mr Paton was concerned that his partner was planning to have a termination and that he had no rights to be consulted about this, or to prevent it taking place. He took the case to court. In 1978, the court found that in law there is no right of veto over a termination by a father, whether or not he is married to the woman. The court found in law that the father is not even entitled to information about an impending termination.

Mr Paton took his case to the European Court of Human Rights and argued that he should have a right to prevent the termination taking place because Article 2 provides a protection of law to the right to life. The European Court of Human Rights found that the Convention right did not prevent abortion taking place. The right to life in the foetus could not be held to be more important than the right of the mother.

Paton v *BPAS* (1978) and *Paton* v *UK* (1980)

Activity

Write down all the objections you have heard against termination on moral grounds. Then write down all the arguments you have heard in favour of termination. These do not have to match what you yourself believe about abortion. Can you identify from this other areas of moral debate that have not been discussed above?

Legal accountability

The law has had to create a framework that takes account of the ethical views held by society. The Abortion Act 1967 (amended in 1990) provides that a termination can take place within the first 24 weeks of pregnancy but only for one of a defined set of reasons, and then only with the agreement of two doctors who believe these reasons are in good faith. Nurses do not have a right to be one of the clinicians deciding that the reason is in good faith because they are not named in the legislation. The Abortion Act assumes that a viable birth can take place after 28 weeks, which is why the limit in the legislation has been set at 24 weeks.

The legislation therefore gives doctors a very wide discretion in deciding whether any of the grounds have been met. This was intended by the Act.

The grounds for termination in the Act are:

- The continuation of the pregnancy would involve risk of injury to the physical or mental health of the pregnant woman or any of her existing children.

- The termination is necessary to prevent grave permanent injury to the physical or mental health of the woman.
- The continuation of the pregnancy would involve risk to the life of the pregnant woman.
- There is a substantial risk that the child would suffer from such physical or mental abnormalities as to be seriously handicapped.

The law has never given rights to the protection of an unborn foetus. The law only provides protection when the child is born.

There are now legal protections for this right of conscientious objection. These are set out in the Abortion Act 1967 which provides a right of conscientious objection to those who would be involved in a procedure of termination. This means that there is a legal protection for individuals who wish to assert this ethical right. The legal framework provides that this protection does not apply where the involvement of the individual clinician would be 'necessary to save the life or prevent grave permanent injury to the pregnant woman'. This would suggest that if a woman had been admitted to hospital for a termination and then had a heart attack, the nurse on the ward would not be able to rely on the conscientious objection clause to avoid providing care.

The Abortion Act 1967 only allows a doctor to carry out a termination under section 1(1). It was unclear whether a nurse or other health professional could carry out procedures to induce the termination, and this point was considered in the courts. The ruling was that such procedures were allowed by the legislation.

Case study 11.2: RCN seeks clarification of guidance for nurses

In the case of *RCN* v *DHSS* (1981), the Royal College of Nursing went to the House of Lords to seek clarification of guidance that had been issued by the DHSS. This guidance set out the ways that a nurse could be involved in adjusting the flow of prostaglandin and oxytocin through a drip valve and adding fresh supplies of both as necessary. The RCN wanted clarification of whether this was contrary to section 1(1) of the Abortion Act 1967. The House of Lords considered each step that a nurse would be involved in as a result of the guidance, and compared this with their interpretation of section 1(1). They found that the nurse's involvement did not breach this section and that the guidance was therefore consistent with the legislation.

Activity

Do you consider that nurses should have the legal right stated in the Abortion Act 1967 to decide whether the reason given for the termination is given in good faith? What are your reasons for this?

Employment accountability

Because the use of the conscientious objection in relation to abortion is now included in law, employers have to respect this right when it is used by a member of staff. Some pressure may be exerted on an individual staff member by her colleagues not to exercise this right. It is important for nurse managers to make it clear to staff that this right exists, and allow for a discussion on how it may be used.

As the care of individuals seeking fertility or termination treatment is specialised, it is likely that the nurse will know in advance whether she wants to work in this area. The contract of employment may provide that the nurse works in areas that deal with termination or fertility, and local protocols may set out the methods to be used if other colleagues want to exercise their right to conscientious objection.

Activity

Imagine that one of your colleagues tells you she has a conscientious objection to abortion. How would you help her share this with her team?

Commentary on scenario

Patricia will need to be aware of the following:

Professional
She may voice a conscientious objection and rely on the NMC Code of Professional Conduct, but she would not be able to leave the health care setting until she was sure that alternative arrangements had been made. She should therefore ask the agency to find someone else to take over her shift, and remain there until that person arrives. If the agency cannot find someone else, the NMC may feel Patricia has broken the Code if she just leaves the clinical situation.

Ethical
Patricia's views have a moral grounding, and the value of this is reflected in law and in professional guidance. She may not have known that her values were so strong in this area, until she was faced with working in that clinical situation. Now that she does know, she will be able to make sure that her conscientious objection is recorded with the agency in relation to further work with them.

Legal
The law allows a conscientious objection to be raised under the Abortion Act 1967. The Act does not require that the nurse has to stay on duty until alternative arrangements have been made, so the NMC Code

is drafted more tightly in relation to the response expected of a nurse. However, the law allows conscientious objection to the 'participation' in a termination. It does not extend this right of objection to providing care to the woman either before or after the procedure. If the ward were a recovery ward, the legal right would not allow Patricia simply to walk away.

Employment

Patricia does not have a contract of employment with the hospital. She has been asked to work there by the agency. She needs to let the ward sister know immediately that she has a problem working on this ward, but stay there until alternative arrangements can be made to ensure there is adequate nursing staff. She needs to let the agency know that she should not be asked to cover this type of clinical setting in the future, and to make sure that she checks this every time she is offered an agency shift. Depending on whether another member of staff can be found, she should negotiate with the agency whether she is paid for the hours that she attended the ward.

Palliative care and gifts

Sensitivity of nurses who are involved in palliative care is needed not just to ensure that the health needs of the patient are met, but that the individual recognises that he or she is dying. This also calls for recognition of the greater family dynamic and the different reactions by family members to proposed treatment.

The vulnerability of patients at the end of their life has a further dynamic which can affect nursing practice, and that involves the desire on the part of the patient to make some recognition of the value placed on that care. In some extreme cases, this may mean the patient leaves a gift to the nurse or to the hospice or health setting in which the care was provided.

The horror of the events surrounding the activities of Harold Shipman, a GP who was found to have deliberately ended the lives of his patients, has raised wider questions in society about the nature of trust in the clinical relationship at such a vulnerable time.

This section considers the complex issue of providing skilled palliative care where the patient tells the nurse that a gift is being left in the will.

Scenario

Christiana is an experienced palliative care nurse. She has been caring for a patient called Simon who has multiple sclerosis and is now very weak. Simon has been told that he has only a few days to live. Simon has no close family. He is not married and does not have a partner. His mother has died and his father has moved to Australia to live with Simon's sister.

As Simon's condition worsens, his pain increases. The doctor prescribes medication and Christiana administers this. Simon tells Christiana that he has made a will in which he has left his house in Bath to her.

Christiana continues to care for Simon but in her break she makes an appointment to see her manager to discuss the decision by Simon to leave her property in his will. She wonders what her accountability is in this situation. The issues she will need to address are set out below under each pillar of accountability, followed by a commentary on the scenario.

Professional accountability

The NMC Code of Professional Conduct has a short clause that deals with the provision of gifts to a nurse. Clause 7.4 states 'You must refuse any gift, favour or hospitality that might be interpreted, now or in the future, as an attempt to obtain preferential consideration.'

This is not restricted to gifts from patients but is wide enough to cover gifts from family members, pharmaceutical or other commercial companies, or private sector organisations. The key issue being addressed by the NMC is not in relation to the gift itself, but it focuses on the way that the gift might be interpreted by others. The advantage of this clause is that a nurse does not have to refuse out of hand a token of appreciation that is given by the family or the patient in the context of the relationship.

It is important to bear in mind that the interpretation of the gift may take place at some point in the future. This means that there may be scrutiny of the gift even after the clinical relationship has ended.

The main objection to receiving a gift, for the NMC, is that this may have a detrimental impact on the clinical relationship; the key phrase is 'preferential consideration'. It is therefore crucial for the nurse to consider, whenever she or he is presented with a gift, or the promise of a gift, to assess whether this may be linked in any way with preferential consideration. This phrase is not defined by the NMC.

The Department of Health has published guidance for nurse prescribers who receive gifts from pharmaceutical companies (Department of Health, 2003). This states that 'as part of the promotion of a medicine or medicines, suppliers may provide inexpensive gifts and benefits, for example pens, diaries or mouse mats. Personal gifts are prohibited, and it is an offence to solicit or accept a prohibited gift or inducement. Companies may also offer hospitality at a professional or scientific meeting or at meetings held to promote medicines, but such hospitality should be reasonable in level and subordinate to the main purpose of the meeting.'

Activity

The nurses on a paediatric ward are used to receiving boxes of chocolates from parents who want to express their thanks for the nursing care provided. When the father of a young boy with leukaemia turns up one day with a plasma television for use in the staff room, there is some discussion over whether this gift can be accepted. The child has only recently been diagnosed and will require further ongoing treatment from the staff.

What would you say are the arguments for and against taking this gift?

Ethical accountability

There are people who may be aware they have a terminal condition but do not want information about this. It is important that staff are aware of the extent to which the person can receive that information. There are also issues concerning the involvement of the family. This is particularly difficult where the patient expresses wishes about his or her death that are not consistent with what the family would want to happen. The dilemma for the nurse is that where the patient's family want to know but the patient refuses to give consent for the information to be passed on, giving the information to the family may be a breach of confidence even though it may assist the family member in the dying process.

Those who are in favour of euthanasia argue that promoting autonomy involves giving everyone a right to die. Those who are against euthanasia argue that there are concerns at the potential for influence from family members on an individual who may feel that he or she has become a burden to the family or to society.

The ethical principles in acts and omissions have been considered in Chapter 3 in greater detail. The debate is whether failing to intervene, omitting to act, is an appropriate ethical response where the individual autonomy of an individual is concerned. There is no moral criticism for a person who did not come to the rescue of another in distress because there is no moral imperative that demands intervention in another person's life. However, where an individual does act to intervene, the action can be criticised. Where a person is dying, therefore, the ethical standard is that there is no criticism on the part of the nurse for failing to keep someone alive. However, there is criticism where the nurse actively takes part in causing death.

Legal accountability

Most decisions about the type of treatment and care that should be given to an individual who is dying can be made by doctors and nurses based on their professional judgement. Nurses who are expert in palliative care will be attuned to the very slight changes in pallor and breathing that can give an idea about how much longer a person has to live. This expert clinical care is relied upon to ensure that the appropriate care is given to the patient in relation to pain relief, skin care and hydration. It is important that the nurse acts in accordance with the body of professional opinion about the care to be given in order to be sure that the legal standard (the Bolam test) is reached.

Because the ethical issues in relation to death and dying are so intricate, where there are issues to be raised about the legal aspects of a proposed treatment, a very effective legal device has been used by Trusts, individual family members or members of the health care team. This is known as a *declaration.* It involves going to court to seek legal approval that a proposed action will not be unlawful. The key areas of law that arise in the context of the care of the dying relate to murder and manslaughter. It is a criminal offence to take an action that results in the death of another person.

Case study 11.3: Seeking a declaration to withdraw artificial hydration and nutrition

The most famous case on this point was *Airedale NHS Trust* v. *Bland.* Tony Bland was a young football supporter who was crushed at the Hillsborough Football Stadium in 1989. He was diagnosed with persistent vegetive state (PVS) and the prognosis was that he would never recover from this. He was being given artificial hydration and nutrition. His family and the health care team wanted to withdraw this artificial hydration and nutrition but were concerned that this might be regarded in criminal law as manslaughter. They went to the House of Lords for a declaration in advance that the proposed withdrawal of the treatment would be lawful. The court approved, so the withdrawal went ahead.

Airedale NHS Trust v. *Bland* (1992)

Where the individual does not consider the consequences of his or her action in relation to the death of a patient, the law may prosecute the individual for murder (intentional and premeditated killing of another) or for manslaughter (unintentional killing of another).

The European Convention on Human Rights will protect the legal process over the right to life in Article 2, but will stop at providing that all life must be preserved at all cost because of the provisions in Article 3 which prohibit inhuman and degrading treatment. Where an individual is being resuscitated and is very frail, there will be a point at which the provisions of Article 3 could be used to argue that aggressive treatment outweighs the dignity of the individual.

Case study 11.4: High dosage resulting in murder trial

Dr Cox was found guilty of attempted murder for giving a very high dose of potassium chloride to a patient who was dying. The amount in the dose caused her death. The evidence at the trial was that there were no pain relieving properties in the drug and Dr Cox knew that the amount he was giving would result in death.

R v. Cox (1992)

Employment accountability

There is no law that can prevent a nurse from being a witness to a will but there may be local policy from the employer on this. Therefore, it is always worthwhile checking the current policies of employers. It is important to note that where a nurse is a witness to a will, he or she cannot be a beneficiary or obtain a bequest from the will. It is also important to note that in the event that a will is disputed, the people who witnessed the signing of the will can be later drawn into litigation. Most employers therefore do not encourage nurses to be a witness to a will in the course of their employment. It would be more desirable and appropriate for someone else who is independent and forthcoming to undertake the task. Some employers appoint this task to specific people, usually managers, in the workplace.

Health Service Guidance (Department of Health, 1993) sets out steps which are aimed primarily at maintaining standards of business conduct and preventing corruption in the award of contracts. It does however offer guidance on casual gifts from relatives and patients and states: 'Articles of low intrinsic value such as diaries or calendars, or small tokens of gratitude from patients or their relatives need not necessarily be refused. In cases of doubt staff should either consult their line manager or politely decline acceptance.'

Most settings in which palliative care is provided will have policies that provide ways of dealing sensitively with the issue of gift giving and the bequests that may be made by patients in their wills.

Commentary on scenario

Christiana will need to be aware of the following:

Professional

She has been told that she is to be left a gift by the patient. She will need to consider whether any interpretation could be placed on this by anyone else, particularly after Simon dies. Christiana will need to consider that others may want to investigate whether the gift was related in any way to the care that she gave Simon. If there is even a remote possibility that this may be the case, she should contact the NMC in writing and set out the information she has been given. This is to ensure that her personal professional accountability with the NMC is maintained. In the event that a concern is raised through the fitness to practice procedures, the letter will demonstrate that Christiana considered her professional accountability in an informed manner, and took action on this.

Ethical

The ethical issues will involve the need for Christiana to make an assessment of whether the gift is to be perceived as an attempt to ask for future personal care and attention, which may go beyond the level of independent and professional care that would normally be provided. Because she has been told that a large gift has been promised to her, she will need to assess how far this alters the balance in the nurse–patient relationship. The more insidious consequence would be if it may be perceived that she has taken any action that may hasten death in order to obtain the bequest. Any nursing care that would involve adjusting amounts of pain-relieving medication, for example, may be scrutinised to see whether a motive other than nursing care in the best interests of the patients may exist. Because the bequest can only come to Christiana after the patient has died, it would raise questions about any form of care she gave or requested for him that may be interpreted as influencing or hastening his death. For these two reasons, on ethical grounds, it may be appropriate for Christiana to consider whether she should withdraw from providing direct care to the patient.

Legal

Because the patient has said this is being left in his will, there are certain legal rules that will apply. When the patient dies, his possessions and debts are counted, and the balance of his estate is then distributed according to the terms of his will. It is always possible to refuse to receive a bequest in a will. There is no rule that prevents a nurse from receiving a gift in a will unless the will is challenged for its overall legality. This may occur if there was a doubt about the mental capacity of the patient at the time the will was made. It may also occur if there was an allegation of duress or undue pressure being placed on the patient by the healthcare professional at the time the will was made. Christiana should make a very full note of the conversations she has with the patient about this, so that if there is an investigation about the will, she can be clear about the first time that she became aware the bequest had been mentioned. She is not under any obligation to discuss this with any family members.

Employment

Christiana knows that the patient has informed her about a bequest in a will. It would be sensible for her to inform her managers of this. She is not under an obligation to say what the bequest is. Because she is still providing nursing care to the patient, she will need to discuss whether the knowledge of the bequest means that she should withdraw from providing him with direct care. This would enable Christiana and her manager to be sure that they have taken active steps to ensure that no undue influence will affect future nursing decisions made by Christiana. If Christiana does not notify her managers, she may be in breach of the implied contractual term of trust and confidence. This may lead to the disciplinary process being used. She should also find out whether her employer has a policy in relation to the acceptance of gifts and bequests in order to be sure the she follows any notification processes. Her managers cannot demand that she refuse the bequest. Christiana should document every meeting that she has with her managers on this issue so that a proper audit trail exists.

Conclusion

This chapter has set out some specific scenarios that relate to all four pillars of accountability. The intention is to demonstrate that this framework can be used in complex areas of nursing practice. Each nurse can adopt this framework to use in answering questions about the extent and the boundaries of his or her accountability in any setting. While all the details may not be immediately apparent, it provides the basis on which the nurse can be sure that he or she has considered the appropriate questions.

The function of this text has been to set out an approach to accountability with a framework for nursing practice that encourages critical evaluation and leads to greater confidence, even where the complexity of the nursing situation may be sensitive. Patients will benefit from being cared for by nurses who have this assurance about their practice, and the trust needed in that clinical relationship will be reinforced across the whole of the profession.

By now, you should be able to:

- apply the four pillars of accountability in complex areas of health care
- understand where to access further information for each pillar of accountability in your nursing practice
- be confident that the four pillars of accountability apply to any nursing situation.

Useful websites

Royal College of Obstetricians and Gynaecologists: www.rcog.org.uk
Information on making a will: www.thewillsite.co.uk

If you need to find a solicitor, visit the Law Society's website www.solicitors-online.com for a searchable list of over 80 000 registered solicitors.

References

Abortion Act 1967. The Stationery Office, London.

Airedale NHS Trust v. *Bland* (1993) 1 All ER 341.

Department of Health (1993) *Standards of Business Conduct for NHS Staff*. Health Service Guidance (93)5. The Stationery Office, London.

Department of Health (2003) *Gifts and Benefits from Suppliers of Medicines*. DoH, London.

House of Commons Social Services Committee (1989–1990) *Abortion Act 1967 'Conscience Clause'*. HC paper 123.

Nursing and Midwifery Council (2002) *Code of Professional Conduct*. NMC, London.

Paton v. *BPAS* (1978) 2 All ER 987.

Paton v. *UK* (1980) 3 EHRR 408.

RCN v. *DHSS* (1981) 1 All ER 545.

RCOG (2004) *The Care of Women Requesting Induced Abortion – Evidence-based Clinical Guideline Number 7*. Royal College of Obstetricians and Gynaecologists, London.

R. v. *Cox* (1992) 12 BMLR 38.

Index